Active Ageing, Active Learning

EDUCATION IN THE ASIA-PACIFIC REGION: ISSUES, CONCERNS AND PROSPECTS

Volume 15

For further volumes:
http://www.springer.com/series/5888

Gillian Boulton-Lewis • Maureen Tam
Editors

Active Ageing, Active Learning

Issues and Challenges

Springer

Editors
Gillian M. Boulton-Lewis
Queensland University of Technology
Brisbane, Queensland
Australia
gillianbl@bigpond.com

Maureen Tam
The Hong Kong Institute of Education
Tai Po
Hong Kong SAR
China
msltam@ied.edu.hk

ISBN 978-94-007-2110-4 e-ISBN 978-94-007-2111-1
DOI 10.1007/978-94-007-2111-1
Springer Dordrecht Heidelberg London New York

Library of Congress Control Number: 2011938283

Printed on acid-free paper

Springer is part of Springer Science+Business Media (www.springer.com)

Series Editors' Introduction

One of the most striking features of the modern world is its changing demographic profile. In almost any policy arena, the issue of demographic change (or ageing) sits alongside globalisation, climate change and the knowledge revolution as areas which are transforming societies, including the ways in which we organise and go about our work activities. This is a significant and worldwide phenomenon. What emerges is a picture of a worldwide trend that touches many aspects of, for example, employment and the labour market, but one which also needs to take account of the very different economies, political systems and societies in the world.

The scale of this demographic change means that ageing is no longer a matter of how individuals adapt to the ageing process but how society adapts to the irreversible changes that are under way. In many countries, current policies and institutions are not designed to address the challenges and opportunities of this future, either in terms of education or the world of work. Looking at Asia, Japan has nearly 23% of the population over 65 years old and for the last 3 years has had negative population growth. Thailand has over 9% aged over 65 but has a population growth rate of approximately 0.6% pa. Taiwan has 10% aged over 65 and has a growth rate that has declined from 0.64% pa in 2000 to 0.23% in 2009. Hong Kong has 12.5% aged over 65, and it is estimated that this will rise to 26.8% by 2033. It also has one of the lowest population growth rates in the world.

A common perception is that an ageing population will have negative consequences for society. We regularly hear alarm bells sounding from governments, particularly in the developed world, about the financial consequences in terms of increased pension, health and care costs and the social consequences through the requirement for additional family care responsibilities and an increased tax base for the ever decreasing working population. Reactions in certain countries have been to consider raising the retirement age, or more accurately, to raise the age at which state pension provisions and other benefits for the elderly will be provided. This is not proving a politically popular option in many countries, especially amongst those people who are approaching retirement age or those that have physically demanding jobs. Singapore has introduced 'from retire to rehire' as a policy measure. This provides retraining for elderly employees who are approaching retirement age or who have retired and wish (through desire or necessity) to return to the labour force.

What has not actually been proven conclusively is how much actual concrete evidence justifies these government reactions to ageing. We do not fully understand, for example, how changes in the age structure of the population will affect social attitudes, values, norms and behaviours. There is much uncertainty over social and economic variables. Knowledge is continuing to be developed through research into the impact of population ageing, and the contributors to this book provide valuable research and insight to address the key questions that are raised by an ageing population:

- How can a large elderly population that is living longer maintain its productivity and contribute to its own and society's well-being?
- Will an ageing population change the economies, cultures and politics?
- How can institutions and policies related to workforce development and health-care and education be reformed to positively affect the future?
- Will an ageing population widen the gap between the haves and have-nots?
- How will continued learning contribute to active ageing and a healthier lifestyle for people as they age?

Education is going to become increasingly important in an ageing world to enable people, in particular those with physically demanding work, to gain new workplace skills to enable them to work for longer as retirement ages are edged upwards in response to increased longevity.

This book provides a fascinating collection of papers that discuss the issues involved and highlights the dedication and the commitment of the authors in this volume in the field of elderly learning.

Tokyo, Japan — Ryo Watanabe
Hong Kong SAR, China — Rupert Maclean

Foreword

Many countries throughout the world are facing the prospect of a rapidly ageing population over the present and forthcoming decades – with quite radical shifts in the age profiles of their populations. This demographic phenomenon is arising from a complexity of social, economic, aspirational, health and medical factors, resulting in both falling birth rates and higher levels of longevity. It is presenting countries with the demographic reality and continuing prospect of diminishing proportions of citizens of normal working age and increasing proportions of elderly. It is challenging life-stage traditions in which participation in the workforce is seen as ending shortly before a generally short period of retirement in relative passivity and declining health and ability. It is also challenging social services, governments, economic planners, families and individuals with imperatives to review their own understanding and expectations of older persons and the established practices that they have in relation to the elderly.

Prominent among the social service institutions thus affected is that of education, especially from a lifelong learning perspective. A rapidly ageing population underlines the imperative to see educational opportunities and learning engagements distributed throughout the lifespan. It highlights the economic, health and welfare benefits of active learning in older age. It makes nonsense of stereotypes of older persons as non-adaptive, non-learners, fixed in their ways.

Prominent among the countries facing these realities is the Peoples' Republic of China and its Hong Kong Special Administrative Region – the former particularly through the success of its central family planning directives, the latter as the consequence of its advanced economic and social status.

Responding to that context, the Hong Kong Institute of Education has established a Centre for Lifelong Learning Research and Development with a particular focus on elderly learning, through its Elder Academy. An early focus of that Academy was to commission a series of critical reviews to evaluate the issues, policies, research and practices internationally in elderly learning and education. Those reviews – undertaken by a selection of internationally renowned researchers and scholar-practitioners in the field – were designed both to inform its own research and development plans and its advice to government instrumentalities in Hong Kong and elsewhere. They were commissioned both for formal public presentation through a seminar series in Hong Kong and for international publication, in order to make them more widely available to educational planners, policy makers, providers and concerned members of the public worldwide.

This volume satisfies that latter goal in making a scholarly, informed and critical but very readable and practically grounded set of contributions available to an international readership. The initial set of seminar papers has been here supplemented by others commissioned to further enrich the overall picture of the field.

Deputy Dean (Research)
Convenor, Doctor of Education Program
School of Education and Professional Studies
(Brisbane, Logan)
Faculty of Education Mt. Gravatt campus
Griffith University, Australia

Professor Richard G. Bagnall

Preface

This book provides a unique collection of chapters by authors who are committed to supporting learning by elders internationally and in Hong Kong specifically. It focuses on ageing and learning, describes why learning is so important throughout life, attempts to counter ageism as it affects thinking about learning by elders and others in the community, presents some research in ageing and implications and describes provisions for ageing and learning in some parts of the Asia Pacific region.

The book arose from a series of seminars on Elder Learning, organized by Professor Richard Bagnall, then Director of the Centre for Lifelong Learning Research and Development, which took place at the Elder Academy of the Hong Kong Institute of Education from January to March 2009. The seminars were sponsored by the Elderly Commission and the Labour and Welfare Bureau of Hong Kong. The Foreword by Bagnall explains the origin of the seminars. The unifying theme of the seminars was ageing and learning. The intention was to provide background on issues for learning by elders in Hong Kong. The series included invited presentations dealing with lifelong learning, welfare and mental well-being into older age (Field, 09/01/2009); international educational initiatives for the elderly (Swindell, 16/01/2009); a narrative of learning and longevity (Pfahl, 20/02/2009); education for the elderly: why, how and what? (Boulton-Lewis, 06/03/2009); and Chinese ageism lives on: grassroots reports on elderly learning in rural Shaanxi, Jiangxi and Jiangsu (Boshier, 20/03/2009). To complement the seminars, there are additional invited chapters from Chui, Buys and Miller, Biggs and Tam. Chui describes and compares elderly learning in four different Chinese communities. Buys and Miller discuss the development of a quantitative multidimensional measure of active ageing. Biggs applies critical narrativity to stories of ageing in social policy, and Tam describes policy and support for lifelong learning by seniors in Hong Kong.

This compilation of scholarly work should constitute a valuable recent resource to contribute to the global understanding and knowledge base for later life learning and elder education.

Preface

[illegible]

Contents

Chapter 1
Introduction

Gillian M. Boulton-Lewis

The book contains perspectives on the worldwide phenomenon of ageing and its implications, on reasons why elders should keep on learning, on provisions for learning and ageing, ways to measure implications of policies for ageing and active ageing and finally ageing and learning in the Asia Pacific region, including China, other parts of Asia and Hong Kong. It presents and discusses therefore a range of recent issues and perspectives on ageing and learning and should constitute a valuable recent resource for anyone involved in education for elders in Hong Kong, in particular, and elsewhere in Asia. There is some overlap in the issues raised in the chapters, as is to be expected when a series of people are asked to address learning and ageing from different perspectives; however, there is no disagreement about the benefits and need for elders to be assisted to keep learning.

The chapters have been organized into three sections. The first section, concerned with ageing issues and provisions for learning, includes the chapters by Field, Boulton-Lewis and Swindell. The next section, including the chapters by Pfahl, Biggs and Buys and Miller, is concerned with some research methods on ageing issues. The final section focuses on provisions for ageing in parts of Asia and Hong Kong and includes chapters by Boshier, Chui and Tam.

The phenomenon of ageing worldwide, its implications generally and the need and provisions for learning as vital to active ageing are addressed by various authors. Statistics that illustrate what some have called the 'silver tsunami' and its likely social, economic and cultural implications are presented from different perspectives by Field, Boulton-Lewis and Swindell. Field focuses on learning, welfare and mental well-being in older age and includes an overview of the profound changes that have taken place during older adults' lives. The complex consequences of global ageing

G.M. Boulton-Lewis (✉)
Queensland University of Technology, Brisbane, QLD, Australia
e-mail: gillianbl@bigpond.com

G.M. Boulton-Lewis and M. Tam (eds.), *Active Ageing, Active Learning: Issues and Challenges*, Education in the Asia-Pacific Region: Issues, Concerns and Prospects 15,
DOI 10.1007/978-94-007-2111-1_1, © Springer Science+Business Media B.V. 2012

and the policy challenges they present for countries worldwide are discussed. Field points out that many older people are choosing to stay in the workforce, and hence, there is a blurring in the age of retirement and the need for a new understanding of ageing. Field also notes that despite the apparent benefits of continued learning there is a decline in participation with age.

Much of the anxiety about ageing populations, evidenced by governments, is due to the costs of care and health provisions for the elderly at the expense of younger members of the population. However, recent research points to the significant role that lifelong learning can play in promoting mental well-being and resilience and preventing cognitive decline in ageing. There is limited empirical evidence, still mostly correlational, that education in early life or in ageing will halt the decline of cognitive powers. However, it will at least keep older people involved in enjoying and living life fully. It should assist with self-confidence and coping strategies, in maintaining cognitive functioning and knowledge, in health management, keeping up with technology developments, maintaining social relationships and encouraging wisdom. It may even improve neuroplasticity, support new neural pathways and utilize new brain cells (Boulton-Lewis, Swindell, Pfahl). Swindell claims, on the basis of the successful ageing model from the MacArthur Study, an extensive multidisciplinary research project in America, that the fundamental attributes of a successfully ageing individual are: being at low risk of disease and disease-related disability, having high mental and physical function and active engagement with life. These are all interrelated. Maintaining high cognitive functioning is a priority for successful ageing. If the brain is not functioning effectively, other activities are not possible. Learning by people as they age should contribute to independence and self-reliance, reduce social and financial costs of caring and allow elders to continue to contribute meaningfully to society (Boulton-Lewis, Field, Swindell, Pfahl). Boulton-Lewis argues that money invested in active ageing leads to improved health and self-sufficiency and hence reduces costs for governments. Because in recent years there has been a sharp reduction in public provision of recreational education for older adults in Britain, and very little in Australia and most other countries, many older people are turning to the private sector, for example, U3A as described below, reading groups and commercial providers, to meet their needs (Field, Swindell, Boulton-Lewis). Field points out that these opportunities are likely to attract better educated and more affluent elders and neglect the less fortunate. Hong Kong and some other parts of Asia are an exception, and governments are dealing with ageing partly by providing opportunities for active learning by elders.

As a consequence of the poor support for lifelong learning by government and policy makers and the emphasis being on upgrading skills so that older workers can remain in the workforce, a large number of alternative learning initiatives have prospered (Swindell, Boulton-Lewis, Field). The learning opportunities for older learners in a number of countries, by groups described loosely as U3A, are presented in some detail by Swindell. He describes the two alternative U3A models: the French one, mainly sited in universities; and the British one, which is largely a self-help organization. Other approaches have evolved from these models and proliferated in many countries with a range of operations of U3As in Australia, New Zealand,

China and other countries. U3As worldwide incorporate most of the elements for successful ageing and usually include intellectually, physically and socially stimulating learning options prepared and conducted by retired people. Some programmes emphasize skills acquisition, some provide 'catch-up' opportunities and many others focus mainly on the intrinsic value of learning for its own sake. It is suggested that individuals through these groups can influence their own active ageing and transform the stereotypical views which include poor health, decline and dependence because they allow active engagement with life, social networks and the opportunity to do interesting things.

Ageism is evident in most societies but manifests itself in different ways. In the UK and Australia, it is apparent in the lack of government support for learning for elderly citizens (Field, Boulton-Lewis, Biggs). Biggs also discusses ageism in the UK from the perspective of social policy. In rural China, it is strong according to Boshier. Swindell cites work by Harper (2008) who noted that mental development, brain capacity and longevity are closely associated and that unfortunately, UK government policy has tended to equate ageing with large numbers of older people rather than large numbers of people who are just living longer, many of them leading active healthy lives. It is critical that demeaning stereotypes of ageing are challenged and that we accept a new perspective on ageing and learning in modern society. This should focus less on economics and more on quality and continuity of life for all (Field, Boulton-Lewis) and capitalize on older citizens' cognitive resources. It is true that older adults usually experience some decline in physical and cognitive capacities and a risk of social isolation and ill health (Field, Boulton-Lewis) and that educational participation falls with age and reaches very low levels among older adults. Nevertheless, Boulton-Lewis asserts that older people want to keep on enjoying life, participating in society, keeping up with changes and benefiting from problem solving and meaningful activities. Hence, despite age-related decrements in aspects of information processing, we need to focus on what elders can learn and how they might benefit.

The issue of what motivates and assists older adults to keep on learning is important. Boulton-Lewis suggests that sometimes this is in response to life circumstances, or alternatively, it may be due to individual reflection or for continuing self-fulfilment and pleasure. Motivation to learn is also connected with how older people want to learn. Boulton-Lewis claims that as with reasons for learning, how elders want to learn is based on needs and prior experiences and ranges from learning on their own to one-to-one tuition or formal classes. The positive outcomes of seniors researching ageing are also discussed. There is very little research that describes what older people *themselves* say they want and need to learn (Boulton-Lewis); however, there are statements about what others believe is necessary, for example, in health management, finance and use of technology. There is no doubt that we need more data from older people themselves about their attitudes to learning and why, how and what they want to learn. It would also be valuable to have some data about whether such learning has measurable positive benefits.

Boulton-Lewis maintains that use of technology should figure prominently in programmes for practical and cognitive reasons and that studies show that older adults are capable of learning to use technology but are reluctant to do so. Models for promoting its use are discussed. Swindell discusses novel communication technologies in the context of U3A which can cater for people who are isolated by constraints, such as distance or disability; however, confidence is an issue with technology. He describes its important role in helping to maintain the quality of life for older people with its potential to transform aged care and healthcare. He describes courses presented by U3A using aspects of technology and more recently the use of Internet hosted in Australia.

A different perspective on learning and ageing is proposed by Pfahl, who advocates intentional narrative learning for adults. Her focus is on the relationship between learning and longevity fostered by creating narratives to make meaning of experience. She proposes a research-based narrative learning model and discusses its implications for educators and developers addressing learning. The model interprets cognitive and behavioural narrative processes as contributory elements advancing lifelong human learning.

Biggs' work, using narrativity as a method, addresses a critical issue in social policy and ageing, that is, it interrogates political definitions of later life and how these affect older people. The focus is on policies in North America, parts of Europe and the UK. This insightful approach allows the stories that people live by in later life to be made explicit and considered in relation to policy. He asks how social policy and the stories it implies influence the 'spaces' in which we grow old. He believes that thinking in terms of stories allows us to sidestep determinacy and take a stance on other possible positions. He argues that social policy is important because it not only responds to social problems but consecrates and contributes to them. However, policy can also provide visions of experience, such as those in later life, that 'legitimize a space in which social subjects are able to form publicly accepted identities'. A critical assessment of positive ageing policies in the UK suggests at first sight that these are highly facilitative. They challenge ageism as it affects work and access to services and recognize a greater flexibility in lifestyles, income and potential. They support the importance of social inclusion and autonomy for older people. They provide a narrative that is facilitative for people who can finance their own lifestyles or participate in existing social institutions. However, the story in these policies is lacking in alternative pathways for self and social development other than through work or work-like activities. Analysis of the policies raises issues such as: the forms of ageing that are legitimized and delegitimized, how the narratives fit with the social and political experience of older people and whether an inauthentic policy initiative can contribute to spaces for fulfilling ageing.

Buys and Miller describe the development of a quantitative multidimensional measure of active ageing. They assert that, with estimates that two billion of the world's population will be 65 years or older by 2050, ensuring that older people 'age well' is an international priority. To date, however, there is significant disagreement and debate about how to define and measure 'ageing well', with no consensus on either terminology or measurement. They describe an attempt to identify significant contributions to quality of life for older people. They identified eight distinct elements (grouped into four key concepts) which appear to define active ageing: social and life participation (25%), emotional health (22%), physical health and functioning (4%) and security (4%). The intention of their chapter is to prompt informed debate on defining and measuring active ageing and facilitating exploration and understanding of the complex issues that intertwine, converge and enhance the ageing experience.

The chapters by Boshier, Chui and Tam contain recent and unique insights into provisions for active ageing in some parts of the Asia Pacific region. Swindell described a thriving U3A initiative in China, more groups than anywhere else in the world, with some of them supported financially. However, Boshier asserts that this is not reaching into rural areas and that ageism is alive and well in rural China. Chui compares philosophies supporting active ageing in China, Hong Kong, Taiwan and Singapore. The chapters show that opportunities for learning in ageing vary from neglect in rural areas of China to thriving initiatives in urban areas to Confucian beliefs supporting lifelong learning to initiatives in Hong Kong where the motivation is partly to reduce the drain on the economy of the consequences of an ageing population by trying to keep people healthy and independent for as long as possible.

Boshier maintains that Chinese ageism is getting worse. His intention was to analyzed sociocultural impediments to elderly learning in China, give voice to impoverished rural elderly Chinese people and argue the case for offering elderly learners serious intellectual work. He noted that in the Confucian state, older people were venerated, but that this was dramatically eroded by political leaders clinging to power in old age and alienating younger people. It could be that Boshier's findings reflect the fact that his work was undertaken in rural areas where many are illiterate, there is no history of academic activity and where U3As would be difficult to establish. As a result, he maintains that most elderly people in rural China rarely encounter serious intellectual work; are expected to amuse themselves with hobbies, arts, exercise or menial work; and that ageism, human rights and marginalization are prevalent. In rural villages, many mind children while parents work away. He asserts that any serious attempt to build a harmonious society must involve respect for the elderly and determined attempts to foster their learning.

Older adults should not be seen as problems but valued and respected. As active and informed citizens, they are vital to building a harmonious society. Boshier asserts that there are exemplary learning programmes for older adults in China, but a habitual tendency to locate them within formal education inhibits a culture of learning; and too many Chinese officials have prejudicial ideas about elderly persons. Instead of fostering docility, officials should stress active citizenship; there are innovative elements in the national learning initiative, but little is available to senior citizens in rural areas and solutions must reside in communities. People involved with fostering elderly learning in China need arenas wherein they can gather and exchange ideas. Boshier maintains that learning is the heart of addressing nearly every problem in rural China – it could improve health care, environment, economy and other crises. He proposed what might be a template for elderly learning in China in the form of the imaginary Shuang Yu learning village which is committed to making learning the central focus of rural life. Village activists conducted consultations with local people and came up with a learning code which stated that the village was committed to all forms of learning and that everyone should engage in it. A small but energetic group of the fictional Shuang Yu senior citizens felt the last years of life should involve significant learning and possibilities included computers, Chinese art and history, and heritage conservation.

In China, Hong Kong, Taiwan and Singapore, in the Chinese communities, many people still practise and think in a Confucian way, sharing the same Confucian-heritage cultural background from the past. As learning is an essential part of the Confucian culture, it is of interest to determine whether Chinese people with a Confucian background perceive continuation of learning, as they age, differently from each other in the different countries. By elucidating the patterns of elder learning in the four Chinese communities, Chui's chapter explores why and how these older learners pursue lifelong learning, what motivates them to continue to learn and how they would like to be engaged in the learning process. The premise of the comparisons is that their learning approach and behaviour would reflect to some extent the cultural values inherent in each of the four Chinese communities. He also provides a comprehensive picture of the context and provisions for elder learning in the four countries.

In the following chapter, Tam echoes the importance of continued learning to active ageing. She first points out that very little has been said about the impact of cultural influences on elder learning and that no one has discussed learning for and by the elderly across different cultural contexts. Her chapter tries to fill this gap by elucidating the East–West dichotomous view towards lifelong learning by elders in the two different cultural contexts. The chapter then outlines the benefits of continued learning for active ageing and sheds light on a range of learning issues for older learners, including their interests, instructional preferences, facilitators and barriers to participation. In the context of Hong Kong, Tam examines the policies and provisions for elder learning, notes that the Hong Kong government understands that learning is vital to active ageing and has demonstrated this in reports and action, most notably, by setting up the Elder Academy Network to aim at 'education for all ages'. The government has since taken a coordinated approach to later life learning where it is conceived of as an integral part of healthy ageing and is encouraged in the forms of social campaigns, initiatives and even funding support to providers. The Hong Kong government has committed to policies and provided financial support or other resources to help providers run courses and programmes for elders. However, there is limited information as to the effectiveness and impact of such policies and provisions on stakeholders. Tam asserts that there is a critical need for research and evaluation to review the effectiveness, adequacy and the take-up of programmes for and by elders in the Elder Academies.

In summary, the chapters in this book provide considerations of:

- Worldwide population ageing and the implications for learning, welfare and mental well-being in older age
- The reasons, processes and content for learning for the elderly
- Learning opportunities for older learners in a number of countries, all of which can be loosely described as U3A

- Technology in successful ageing and learning
- The relationship between learning and longevity fostered by creating narratives to make meaning of experience
- Narrative analysis of social policy and the need to challenge ageism and other stereotypes
- A quantitative multidimensional measure of active ageing
- Comparisons of opportunities for learning in rural and urban China
- Elder learning in four Chinese communities: China, Hong Kong, Taiwan and Singapore
- Elder education provisions in Hong Kong

Reference

Harper, S. (2008). *Generations and life course: The impact of demographic challenges on education 2010–2050*. Retrieved February 22, 2011, from http://www.ageing.ox.ac.uk/system/files/publication_challenges_on_education_2010–2050.pdf

Part I
Ageing Issues and Provisions for Learning

Chapter 2
Lifelong Learning, Welfare and Mental Well-being into Older Age: Trends and Policies in Europe

John Field

Introduction

Lifelong learning has become an important feature of modern existence. For most policy bodies, lifelong learning is important for mainly economic reasons. In particular, governments have embraced lifelong learning as a way of aligning national education and training systems more closely with other factors that help drive innovation and technological change, with the underlying aim of improving capacities for competitiveness and sustainable growth. The growing significance of lifelong learning for individuals and societies, though, is not solely due to its economic significance. In many nations, there has been a 'silent explosion' in educational participation among adults, as people have increasingly come to see learning – in its many forms – as an everyday part of their lives (Field 2006). This raises important questions for our understanding of learning among older adults.

Survey data consistently show that educational participation falls with age, reaching very low levels among older adults (Aldridge and Tuckett 2008; Schlögl and Schneeberger 2005). This might be important for individual older adults, but since most of them are not in the labour market, it has little wider significance if the main benefits of learning are defined in economic terms. From this human capital perspective, educating older adults has limited benefits even if they are in the labour market because they will not be working long enough to generate adequate returns on the initial investment. Increasingly, though, researchers have started to identify wider social and cultural benefits from participation in learning, and there is also growing evidence of small but important improvements in the mental well-being of individuals. This suggests that older adults can experience significant improvements

J. Field (✉)
School of Education, University of Stirling, Stirling, Scotland
e-mail: john.field@stir.ac.uk

G.M. Boulton-Lewis and M. Tam (eds.), *Active Ageing, Active Learning: Issues and Challenges*, Education in the Asia-Pacific Region: Issues, Concerns and Prospects 15,
DOI 10.1007/978-94-007-2111-1_2,

in quality of life as a result of participating in learning. This paper therefore examines this recent research against the context of older adults' lives and outlines some of the implications for the ways in which we approach learning in later life.

The structure of this chapter reflects the fact that lifelong learning is essentially multifaceted. Adult life is intrinsically social, embedded in relationships and interactions with wide varieties of other people. These relationships and their significance change over time, partly as a result of different life course stages and partly as a result of transformations in many different environments in which people interact with others. Learning is also profoundly cultural in nature. It is influenced by, and in turn influences, the norms and values of the wider community. People's values and attitudes also change over time and therefore affect how they view and engage with different types of learning. And learning is, at the same time, a physical process, which involves the material activities of the brain. Although the brain is shaped by inherited and acquired characteristics of various kinds and can therefore be viewed as partly a social phenomenon, it is also a physical organ whose capacities and processes are highly individual. The chapter therefore examines learning in later life from a range of different perspectives.

The Later Life Course in Context

Contemporary societies are characterized by virtually constant change, and the later phases of life are by no means immune from these powerful trends. Socially, there is a clear tendency towards a 'greying' of the population, as average family sizes decline, the age at which women have their first child gets older and longevity increases among older adults. Second, culturally, there is an increasing tendency for people to consider a range of options in their lifestyles and life choices, and this is having an enormous impact on the family. Some couples choose not to have children at all; some divorce and remarry several times during their lives, and many women choose to return to work soon after having children. This can be seen as part of a wider trend towards what Anthony Giddens refers to as 'institutionalized reflexivity' (Giddens 1991), where all social institutions and practices are subject to scrutiny in the light of constantly changing information. Hence, the continuing debate over what the family is and should be is debated openly and frequently. While this applies to many or even all social institutions, including the informal and formal associations that people access for social support, the family is particularly significant because of its role in providing care for the very young and very old.

Third, there are also significant economic changes. These include growing levels of material comfort for the majority of the population, with many older adults experiencing a rise in average income levels in recent decades (this tendency has been halted in Britain as a result of the financial tsunami, which led to large falls in income derived from investments). This has been accompanied by the growing levels of spending on leisure and lifestyle goods and services, including rising spending on many types of learning activity, from instructional DVDs and videos to study cruises

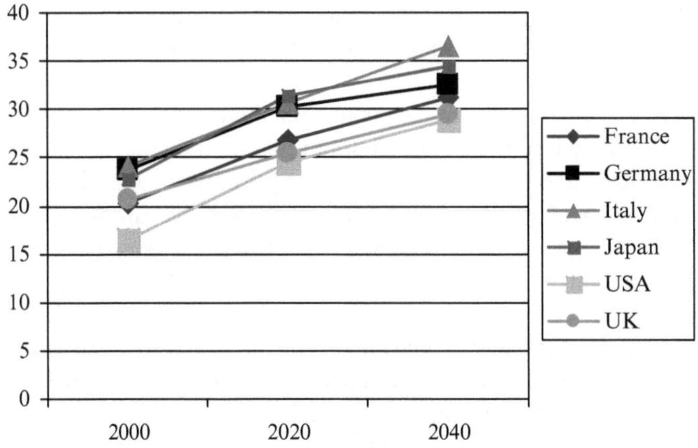

Fig. 2.1 Over-60s as percentage of population (Schuller 2005: 7)

and summer holiday courses. And because of fluctuations in the demand for experienced, skilled and qualified labour, significant numbers of older workers (particularly men in the 50s) have withdrawn from the labour market, whether voluntarily through early retirement or involuntarily through redundancy followed by a period on benefits through to retirement.

These selected examples illustrate some of the profound changes that are taking place in the context of older adults' lives. At the same time, virtually all the industrial societies are ageing. There are different ways of calculating the rise in average ages, but one is particularly significant: namely, the proportion of adults in the population who are at or close to the statutory retirement age. Statutory pensionable ages vary between different countries, and in some countries, they also vary still between men and women. If we simplify matters somewhat, then a quick glance at Fig. 2.1 shows the rapid growth in the number of over-60s as a proportion of the total population in selected industrialized countries. While there are some differences between countries, with Italy (with its low birth rate) at one extreme and the United States (with high immigration) at the other, the upward trend is the same. Within the European Union, it is estimated that by 2020, around one third of the population will be retired, one third will be of working age and one third will consist of young people who have yet to enter the workforce.

This overall trend towards an ageing population is bringing about a considerable growth in the number of adults who are well above the statutory pensionable age. In the United Kingdom, for example, in 2001, the over-75s were 6.4% of the total population; by 2031, it is estimated that they will form 10.6% of the population. Indeed, by 2031, almost 3% of the population will be aged over 85. As well as a 'third age', then, we can speak of a growing proportion of people who will be in their 'fourth age'. And while many, if not all, third agers will continue to lead very active lives, it is inevitable that many of those in the fourth age will experience degrees of cognitive and other physical decline that will constrain their activity levels and may indeed mean that a high proportion will require some kind of care.

As well as an overall ageing of the population, there are also a number of complex social and economic trends that are tending to erode the boundaries between age-related life stages. Among younger adults, changes in the labour market are tending to delay entry into paid employment; in many countries, the vast majority do not take their first full-time job until they are 18 or over. The age at which people first marry is also rising, for both men and women, and men are increasingly likely to live in the parental home until their mid- or late 20s (and even, as in Italy, into their early 30s). Among older adults, far fewer people are retiring at or near to the date at which they reach pensionable age. This tendency is particularly affecting the affluent, who are also likely to have third-level educational qualifications, so it has become far from unusual for men to graduate in their mid-20s and retire in their early 50s, with a total working life of less than 30 years. Meanwhile, there are some areas where male and female life courses are converging. Although most childcare and eldercare are still undertaken by women, there are also growing areas of caring for men (particularly among older men caring for frail partners). And family sizes are in decline, with a considerable minority opting never to have a child at all, while a growing proportion of women spend much of their adult life in paid employment. While levels of female employment vary enormously, even within Europe, these trends are shared among most industrial nations.

These developments are forcing social scientists to rethink previous ideas about the adult life course (Elder 1975). As well as acknowledging the growing fluidity of boundaries between life stages and the ever more complex relations between male and female life courses, researchers also note that participation in education has become increasingly recurrent. Although 'front-loading' – that is, a strong phase of initial investment during childhood and adolescence – remains the norm, growing numbers of adults in industrial societies return to learning throughout their lives. In many countries, such as Britain and the USA, this includes participation on a highly 'non-normative basis', as where adults re-enter educational phases such as university undergraduate programmes that have been designed primarily for young people. In a highly influential study, which was conceptualized in terms of cohorts rather than generations per se, Gielle and Elder (1998) emphasize the multidirectional nature of life course change. Even in the highly regulated welfare states of northern and western Europe, there is a growing tension between the 'standardized life course' that is associated with entitlement to particular public services (pensions, free education, many types of health care) and the increasing fluidity and pluralization of individual life courses. These trends may be particularly marked in the western industrialized nations, where they are accelerated by and in turn reinforce tendencies towards individualization and biographical reflexivity. It is therefore not yet clear how far these reflections apply to Asian societies, particularly those that are currently in particularly rapid and radical economic and social transitions.

Well-being and Learning in Later Life

The simple image of a greying society turns out to denote a much more complex and multifaceted process of ageing and social change. On the surface, this process looks deeply problematic for societies that have culturally oriented themselves in recent decades towards youth and that depend economically on a regular influx of young people into the workforce. Now, by contrast, it is commonplace for journalists to write of a 'ticking time bomb' (Scherlaeckens 2009: 1), a metaphor designed to emphasize the inevitability of the demographic processes that lie ahead. The metaphor also suggests a destructive force that is scheduled to blow existing assumptions and relationships into the air. Of course, journalists must exaggerate if they are to persuade us – their audience – to read on. Nevertheless, many people seem to assume that an ageing society is something to be viewed with a mixture of anxiety and fear.

Much of this anxiety focuses on the likely costs of caring for an ageing population. There is accordingly a heightened public debate over intergenerational transfers, much of which tends to assume that young people who are in the labour market are productive, while older adults who are out of the labour market consume. In particular, young people pay taxes, while older adults receive pensions and make disproportionate demands on health and other public services. However, as Martin Kohli (2003) points out, this is a one-sided view. Economically, Kohli points the importance of:

- Widespread intergenerational exchanges of help, with grandparents (predominantly women) providing childcare for parents who are working or committed to other activities (see also Mitchell 2008);
- Voluntary financial assistance, such as parental help when couples buy their first house
- Caring for older adults is often provided by other older adults, with both women and men taking on caring roles for frail partners
- Patterns of inheritance, including pre-death transfers designed to avoid paying taxation on larger sums later on

On the basis of German evidence, Kohli argues that net intergenerational transfers on balance favour the young, whereas older adults, overall, are net givers (Kohli 2003).

As well as contributing informal support, many older adults continue to play a part in the formal labour market. Although engagement with the formal labour market declines in many Western societies from the mid-50s onwards, personal preferences and economic requirements are combined to keep some workers in the labour market well after the statutory pensionable age. In 2005, across the European Union, more than 11% of men and over 5% of women aged 65–69 were employed (European Commission 2008: 207). With the declining numbers of young people now entering the labour market, moreover, older adults represent a significant resource for enterprises. And this matches the preferences of a growing number of older workers, who value work as a source of income but also as a source of social recognition and sociability. A recent study in Britain found that four-fifths of workers aged over 50 were interested in continuing to work after 'normal retirement', provided the conditions were suitable (McNair 2005: 32–33). Assuming that labour demand is high in the future, we may therefore anticipate further blurring of the actual age of retirement.

There has also been a lively recent assertion of the positive contributions made by older adults, at least potentially if not always actually. Stereotypes of old age are common in Western societies: popular television programmes often treat older adults as objects of amusement. When an over-60 was elected leader of one of Britain's main political parties, comedians routinely fell back on lazy jibes about walking aids and memory loss, and after a short period in office, he resigned. Challenging such demeaning stereotypes is therefore important. And indeed, there is some evidence that well-being follows something of a U-shaped – or possibly W-shaped – curve with people in their 20s and in their 60s expressing the highest levels of life satisfaction.

Nevertheless, older adults do experience a fall in their physical capacities and are also likely, at some stage, to experience significant cognitive decline. Those who survive into their 70s and 80s are also likely to experience at least one significantly limiting condition. Social isolation is also a risk to well-being. Since Durkheim, social scientists have shown repeatedly that people who are isolated are more likely, all other factors being held constant, to experience periods of depression and other forms of mental ill health than people who are well connected (Field 2008: 63–64). The elderly are especially vulnerable to isolation in Western nations. Solo households are especially common among elderly, and there are also risks of isolation as a result of exclusion from the labour market, or detachment from neighbours or the death of close friends. Physical ill health is also more common with increasing age, placing constraints on some people's abilities to choose their own way of life and daily routines. So, although people in their 70s are likely to report greater subjective well-being than adults in their 40s, people are less likely to report high well-being as they enter the 'fourth age' in their later 70s and in their 80s. Their well-being and resilience are therefore at risk, along with their ability to exercise choice over the circumstances of their lives.

Learning, it has been argued, is an important inhibitor of cognitive decline among older adults (Kirkwood et al. 2008). This assertion rests on some systematically gathered evidence. Qualitative studies suggest that older learners themselves are strongly persuaded of the benefits of their learning (Withnall 2006). More quantitative work does not on the whole deal primarily with older adults as such, but in the absence of contradictory evidence, we can reasonably conclude that in general, the effects of learning are likely to be similar for people from different age groups. There is longitudinal evidence of adult learning's positive cognitive effect on people in their 50s (Hatch et al. 2007). Accredited learning appears to protect individuals against depression, though it seemingly has little or no impact on happiness, and there may be some association (whether causal or not) between depression and leisure courses (Feinstein et al. 2003). Qualitative research, by contrast, suggests that general adult education helps counter depression (Schuller et al. 2004).

Participation in learning does have an impact on adults' levels of life satisfaction, which is an important aspect of well-being (Feinstein et al. 2003), as well as showing gains among learners in optimism and self-rated well-being (Hammond and Feinstein 2006). Finally, a recent German study showed that older adults were the most likely to identify learning something new as an important element in their own subjective well-being (Schleiter 2008).

There is also persuasive evidence that adult learning has positive effects on those personal attributes that are most closely associated with resilience. The most consistent finding in qualitative research and practitioner narratives is that adult learning produces gains in confidence (Tett and Maclachlan 2007: 159). A detailed qualitative investigation of adult literacy, numeracy and host language education in England found that participants identified both social confidence and personal confidence among the most highly valued outcomes of courses (Barton et al. 2007: 111). Additionally, Hammond and Feinstein's longitudinal analysis (2006) found that learners were more likely to report gains in self-efficacy and sense of agency (perceived control over important life choices) than non-learners. There is, then, general agreement among researchers that learning produces greater confidence and self-efficacy and enhances the ability to cope with crises and change across the life course.

This research suggests that learning is potentially very important to the well-being and resilience of older adults. In turn, as well as contributing directly to older people's quality of life, this may also help to maintain independence and self-reliance. While this may itself be valuable in reducing the social and financial costs of caring for older adults, it is probably more important in enabling older adults to continue to contribute to the wider community, whether through paid employment or through more or less formal voluntary activities of various kinds. Since these activities can include contributions to intergenerational learning (Mitchell 2008), this is likely to enhance stocks of human capital overall.

Learning Among Older Adults

Survey evidence consistently shows that older adults show the lowest participation rates in learning. British survey data in 2008, for example, show that only 5% of adults aged over 75, and only 9% of the 65–74 year olds, were learning at the time of the survey; by contrast, over 20% of people aged 35–44 were learning, and 13% among those aged 55–64 (Aldridge and Tuckett 2008: 15). The same survey showed that 57% of over-75s had done no learning whatever since leaving school. A similar pattern emerges with respect to future intentions to learn: over 90% of over-75s thought it likely that they might take up learning in the future, as against 53% of those aged 25–34 (Aldridge and Tuckett 2008: 29). A very similar pattern has been identified in Austria, both in respect of age and participation, and in respect of age and future learning plans (Schlögl and Schneeberger 2005). All in all, then, current participation levels among older adults are considerably lower than would appear desirable, given the evidence above on the effects that learning has on well-being, resilience and quality of life.

Currently, public education policy has a strong focus on investing in initial schooling. A recent report for the British government concluded that a number of factors are inhibiting participation by older adults, with negative consequences for their well-being and mental capital (Government Office for Science 2008: 216). Indeed, in recent years, British education policies have included a sharp reduction in 'recreational' provision for older adults, leading to a steady decline in participation by older age groups (Aldridge and Tuckett 2008). Public provision in Britain, then, has been turned increasingly away from older adults and re-focused on initial investment into children and young people, and this in turn reflects an economics-derived analysis of returns on investment in human capital, as well as a strong desire to tackle socio-economic inequalities among the young. Yet the (presumably unintended) consequences of this strategy in the education policy area are then at odds with other policy goals which are aimed at promoting resilience, independence and quality of life for older adults.

At the same time, many older adults themselves are turning away from public services and towards the private sector to meet different needs (McNair 2009). Voluntary organizations have considerable appeal for this group, but they tend to draw their membership from those who are already well educated. The University of the Third Age is a good example of this trend. While the U3A has different structures and approaches in different European countries, it relies heavily upon self-help and voluntary effort; in the UK, the U3A vigorously maintains its independence from the formal educational sector and relies solely on its own members to provide teaching and other services. It has been a considerable success in most respects and particularly from the point of view of its members, but it is drawn largely from the ranks of retired service class professionals (Huang 2006; Swindell 1993). The same is also true of reading groups, which tend to appeal primarily to older women with well-educated backgrounds.

There has also been rapid growth in commercial provision. Affluent retirees form a ready market for hotels, heritage agencies, travel companies and other bodies who provide study tours, educational cruises, cookery and wine-tasting classes and residential courses. The cost of commercial provision, as well as the typical curricula, means that commercial provision is mainly directed towards the upper, more affluent end of the market. In both cases, I would expect that there are also socio-cultural forms of exclusion at work; this, though, is a speculative judgement if one is informed by research into other leisure activities.

These trends raise obvious questions for policy makers and others concerned with the learning and well-being of older adults. Private provision has proven highly successful in attracting some groups of older adults into learning, but at a price. First, participation is highly stratified on socio-economic grounds. Second, there are issues of quality and focus, particularly in the market for commercial provision. This poses significant risks of market failure combined with increased inequality among the older adult population.

There is no shortage of constructive debate nor of positive proposals for developing new programmes and initiatives (Heidecker and Hechl 2007; McNair 2009; Schuller 2005). Among other priorities for older adults should be:

- Initiatives which combine learning with efforts to maintain and renew social capital
- Engaging older adults in age-appropriate levels of physical activity as a key dimension of learning
- Promoting the use of new technologies as vehicles for learning and sociability among older adults

This is likely to require concerted action across departmental and organizational boundaries since it involves institutions and policy priorities that traditionally lie in different areas. Ultimately, what is required is a new perspective on ageing and learning in modern societies, with a focus less on economic growth and rising consumption, and more on achieving a higher quality of living for all. This in turn may require us to develop a new language of age, which is less easily channelled into derogatory stereotypes and allows us to reconceptualize what it means to be an older adult in a modern society.

References

Aldridge, F., & Tuckett, A. (2008). *Counting the cost: The NIACE survey on adult participation in learning 2008*. Leicester: National Institute for Adult Continuing Education.

Barton, D., Ivanič, R., Appleby, Y., Hodge, R., & Tusting, K. (2007). *Literacy, lives and learning*. London: Routledge.

Elder, G. H. (1975). Age differentiation and the life course. *Annual Review of Sociology, 1*, 165–90.

European Commission. (2008). *The life of women and men in Europe – A statistical portrait*. Luxembourg: Office for Official Publications.

Feinstein, L., Hammond, C., Woods, L., Preston, J., & Bynner, J. (2003). *The contribution of adult learning to health and social capital* (Research Report 8). London: Centre for Research on the Wider Benefits of Learning.

Field, J. (2006). *Lifelong learning and the new educational order*. Stoke-on-Trent: Trentham.

Field, J. (2008). *Social capital*. London: Routledge.

Giddens, A. (1991). *Modernity and self-identity: Self and society in the late modern age*. Cambridge: Polity.

Gielle, J., & Elder, G. (1998). *Methods of life course research: Qualitative and quantitative approaches*. Thousand Island: Sage.

Government Office for Science. (2008). *Mental capital and well-being: Making the most of ourselves in the 21st century*. London: Foresight.

Hammond, C. & Feinstein, L. (2006). *Are those who flourished at school healthier adults? What role for adult education?* (Research Report 17). London: Centre for Research on the Wider Benefits of Learning.

Hatch, S. L., Feinstein, L., Link, B. G., Wadsworth, M. E. J., & Richards, M. (2007). The continuing benefits of education: Adult education and midlife cognitive ability in the British 1946 birth cohort. *Journal of Gerontology, 62*(6), 404–14.

Heidecker, D., & Heckl, E. (2007). *Weiterbildung im alter: Positionen und Perspektiven*. Strobl: Arbeitsgruppe Weiterbildung im Alter.
Huang, C.-S. (2006). The university of the third age in the UK: An interpretative and critical study. *Educational Gerontology, 32*(10), 825–42.
Kirkwood, T., Bond, J., May, C., McKeith, I., & Teh, M.-M. (2008). *Mental capital through life: Future challenges*. London: Government Office for Science.
Kohli, M. (2003). *Generationen in der Gesellschaft, Forschungsgruppe Altern und Lebenslauf* (Forschungsbericht 73). Berlin: Freie Universität Berlin.
McNair, S. (2005). The age of choice: A new agenda for learning and work. In A. Tuckett & A. McAuley (Eds.), *Demography and older learners: Approaches to a new policy challenge* (pp. 27–38). Leicester: National Institute of Adult Continuing Education.
McNair, S. (2009). *Demography and lifelong learning*. Leicester: National Institute for Adult Continuing Education.
Mitchell, W. (2008). The role played by grandparents in family support and learning: Considerations for mainstream and special schools. *Support for Learning, 23*(3), 126–34.
Scherlaeckens, L. (2009, March 11). The age crunch: who's going to be left to do the work in Flanders in 2050? *Flanders Today, 1*, 5.
Schleiter, A. (2008). *"Glück, Freude, Wohlbefinden – welche Rolle spielt das Lernen?" Ergebnisse einer repräsentativen Umfrage unter Erwachsenen in Deutschland*. Gütersloh: Bertelsmann Stiftung.
Schlögl, P., & Schneeberger, A. (2005). *Erwachsenenbildung in Österreich. Hintergrundbericht zur OECD Länderprüfung über Erwachsenenbildung in Österreich*. Wien: Bundesministerium für Bildung, Wissenschaft und Kultur.
Schuller, T. (2005). Demographic challenges: Family structures and ageing. In A. Tuckett & A. McAuley (Eds.), *Demography and older learners: Approaches to a new policy challenge* (pp. 5–25). Leicester: National Institute of Adult Continuing Education.
Schuller, T., Preston, J., Hammond, C., Bassett-Grundy, A., & Bynner, J. (2004). *The benefits of learning: The impacts of formal and informal education on social capital, health and family life*. London: Routledge.
Swindell, R. (1993). U3A (the University of the Third Age) in Australia: A model for successful ageing. *Ageing & Society, 13*(3), 246–66.
Tett, L., & Maclachlan, K. (2007). Adult literacy and numeracy, social capital, learner identities and self-confidence. *Studies in the Education of Adults, 39*(2), 150–67.
Withnall, A. (2006). Exploring influences on later life learning. *International Journal of Lifelong Education, 25*(1), 29–49.

Chapter 3
Issues in Learning and Education for the Ageing*

Gillian M. Boulton-Lewis

Introduction

The world's population is ageing rapidly. According to United Nations statistics, people aged 60 and above made up 11% (705 million) of the world's population in 2007. By 2050, the percentage is expected to double with about 22% (two billion) of the world's population aged 60 years and over (United Nations 2007). In Hong Kong, it is predicted that 28% of the population will be over 65 by 2039 (Hong Kong Population Projections 2010–2039). One in four Australians (25%) will be old (65 years or more) by 2044–2045 (Australian Government Productivity Commission 2005). The ageing phenomenon has been described in colourful term as the silver tsunami (Pew Report 2001, cited in Summer 2007). Ageing has an impact on all aspects of human life, including social, economic, cultural and political domains. Understanding and providing for ageing is therefore a significant issue for the twenty-first century. The World Health Organization (WHO 2002) proposed a model of active ageing based on optimizing opportunities for health, participation and security in order to enhance the quality of life for people as they age. The focus of this chapter is on the education and learning aspect of participation in active ageing.

Two recent studies in Australia have explored the concept of active ageing: the Australian Active Ageing survey (National Seniors Productive Ageing Centre 2005) investigated the indicators and meaning of active ageing for older adults, and the Department for Community Development, Government of Western Australia (2006) developed and implemented the Active Ageing Benchmark Indicators. Both studies described active ageing for older people in terms of being proactive in keeping healthy,

*This chapter is adapted from Boulton-Lewis, G. M. (2009). Education and learning for the elderly: Why, how, what. *Educational Gerontology*, *36*(3), 213–228.

G.M. Boulton-Lewis (✉)
Queensland University of Technology, Brisbane, QLD, Australia
e-mail: gillianbl@bigpond.com

G.M. Boulton-Lewis and M. Tam (eds.), *Active Ageing, Active Learning: Issues and Challenges*, Education in the Asia-Pacific Region: Issues, Concerns and Prospects 15,
DOI 10.1007/978-94-007-2111-1_3,

being physically and mentally active, engaging in learning, living in safe environments, working and actively participating in family and community life. Older adults in the US similarly defined successful ageing as multidimensional including physical, functional, psychological and social health (Phelan et al. 2004). In Britain, Bowling and Iliffe (2006) reported that a multidimensional lay model of ageing predicted quality of life more powerfully than unidimensional models (e.g. biomedical, sociological).

> Stereotypes of decrepit seniors are slowly changing. Today many older adults are described as vibrant and active – they jog, travel, remain socially and politically active, and enjoy learning (Participation Canada 1993). The 21st century should see a new kind of older adult: healthier, better educated and more financially secure (Foot 1996; Martin and Preston 1994)... In the future elders will seek continued personal growth in their retirement years, and hence the demand for educational programmes and services designed to meet the needs of older adults will intensify. Leading adult education researchers agree, "the more education people have, the more education they want, and the more they participate in further learning activities (Cross 1992 cited in Arsenault and Anderson 1998, p. 30.)

Issues in Learning and Ageing

Education and learning are important factors in facilitating participation in society and in allowing adults to enjoy a positive quality of life as they age (WHO 2002, p. 16). Participation within the community is important, firstly, for enjoyment and recreation and, secondly, for allowing older people to adapt to changes within their environment in areas such as technology, lifestyle, finances and health. In addition, the abilities to solve problems and to adapt to change are strong predictors of active ageing and longevity according to Smits et al. (1999). Butler (2002) cites the MacArthur Study on Aging as it confirms that engagement in meaningful activities contributes to good health, satisfaction with life and longevity, as well as reducing the costs of physical and emotional illness.

Learning on its higher forms has been described as understanding, seeing things differently and changing as a person (cf. conceptions of learning as defined by Marton 1988), and this holds at any age. Wolf (2009) proposed four processes of learning: differentiation, dissonance, deconstruction and reconstruction. He illustrated these processes with an example of a 75-year-old woman who had to come to terms with diabetes and learn to make changes in her diet and lifestyle. This challenge, a side effect of ageing, presented her with the need to use all four learning processes. These processes depend on the person's information-processing system functioning adequately – in particular, perception, short-term and working memory and long-term memory. The status of these processes as people age is discussed further below.

Effects of Learning in Ageing

It has been asserted in recent years that learning plays an important role in productive ageing. Lifelong learning and continued education are considered necessary for older people in a society that is characterized by rapid technological changes

(Ardelt 2000). Ardelt contends that it enables elderly people to keep up with technological and scientific advances; to maintain the quality of their lives by enhancing their self-reliance, self-sufficiency and by coping strategies in the areas of physical, health and social relationships; and, in particular, to develop wisdom which requires alternative approaches to learning such as reflection. Dench and Regan (2000) described the effects of formal and informal learning for older people (50 and over) as including enjoyment of life, self-confidence, feelings about self, satisfaction with life, coping ability, increased social involvement and better health. The most important reasons they gave for learning were to keep their brains active and to enjoy the challenge. The most common reasons given for not learning were lack of time and interest. Withnall (2000) noted that recent neurological research shows that mental training in later life can boost intellectual power, assist in maintaining mental function and help to reverse memory decline (Kotulak 1997). Wolf (2009) stated on the basis of substantial research that there is increasing evidence that older adults who are stimulated mentally experience less decline in memory and continued growth in verbal knowledge well into their late seventies.

Ageing and Cognitive Processes

Horn and Hoffer (1992) described nine cognitive processes: (1) knowledge derived from acculturation (M[1]), (2) fluency of retrieval of knowledge (M), (3) visualizing capabilities (M), (4) auditory capabilities (M), (5) quantitative capabilities (M), (6) reasoning capabilities (V[2]), (7) maintaining immediate awareness (V), (8) speed of apprehension (V) and (9) speed of arriving at decisions (V). People high or low on one of these processes are not necessarily high or low in others.

The processes are related in different ways to ageing over the lifespan. Processes which decline late and little in adulthood are said to be maintained (M). Three and 4 increase until forties and then decrease gradually. One, 2 and 5 increase into the sixties before they begin to decline. Individual differences in 1 (knowledge) increase with age because some people continue to learn after formal schooling finishes. The processes 6, 7, 8 and 9 (reasoning, awareness, speed of apprehension and decision making) which decline early in adulthood are considered to be vulnerable (V). They begin to decline slowly from the early twenties. They are also adversely and irreversibly affected by brain damage and can result from small losses in brain functions related to different lifestyles such as consumption of alcohol. Individual differences in 6 do not increase with age. Declines in 6, 7 and 8 result in loss of the ability to comprehend complex relationships. Increases in carefulness and persistence with age to some extent compensate for these losses. Some aspects of 6 improve with training.

Cognitive tests to assess information-processing speed, working memory capability (or short-term memory) and declarative learning, administered to adults aged

[1] Maintained.

[2] Vulnerable.

17–86 years old, found significant age-related decrements in all three constructs (Kirasic et al. 1996).

Recent research focussing specifically on neuropsychological tests to cover cognitive domains that are known to decline as a function of age, including mental speed, several aspects of memory and executive functions, questions the extent of earlier presumed protective effects of higher education on cognitive decline during normal ageing (Van Dijk et al. 2008). They found less decline for older participants who had more education on measures of verbal learning and long-term memory. For measures of interference control, set shifting, semantic and phonemic fluency and mental speed, they found faster decline for individuals with higher age. The Seattle Longitudinal Study (Willis and Schaie 2006) found modest average decline in cognitive function from age 60 to 67 and accelerated decline from 67 to 70 with flatter trajectories in fluid and crystallized intelligence in successive cohorts. This suggests that cognitive functions in the Third Age[3] will become increasingly similar to those in middle age if favourable sociocultural and neurobiological conditions continue. Valenzuela (2009) discussed neuroplasticity and proposed, contrary to earlier thinking, that we continue to develop new brain cells as we age (although they may not be accessible) and that cognitive activity may allow new neural pathways to develop to replace others that have been destroyed.

Much of the research in cognition of older adults as described above is, unfortunately, dominated by identification of obstacles and decline in the process caused by mental and physical deterioration. Ageing is known to affect a number of cognitive processes negatively (Salthouse 1985). It is obvious from research that aspects of the human information-processing system deteriorate with age, in particular, perception, learning and memory processes. However, an outcome of the focus on problem-oriented research on ageing has helped create an image of older people as 'being over the hill, out of date, out of touch, frail, sick and in need of services and support' (Kerschner and Pegues 1998). This picture is compounded by a focus on the effects of diseases, which are more likely with age, that affect physical and social functioning. Declines in cognitive processes should of course be taken into account in designing education for old-old learners (over 75 years in particular). However, it is more useful to take a positive approach and focus on what elders can learn and how they might benefit from such learning.

Older People Can and Do Learn

It is not surprising that older adults want and need to learn – to stay interested in and keep enjoying life to the best of their ability. Wolf (2009) maintained, on the basis of Erikson's model of learning in the eighth stage (Integrality) of development, that education for older persons is also essential for civilization in that it allows them,

[3] Third age: 60–80, fourth age: 80+.

inter alia, to make a contribution to culture based on reflection on their knowledge and experience.

It is known that older adults can and do acquire new knowledge outside of their domains of expertise from earlier learning. Boulton-Lewis (1997) stated that it is clear 'that most adults, as they age usually process less information and do it in a slower and less efficient manner'; however, 'knowledge that has been already acquired, the ability to retrieve it, as well as visual and auditory sensory capabilities are maintained for the most part, into the sixties' at least. Given the time and sufficient motivation, older adults are able to achieve equivalent learning outcomes to younger learners. With extra practice, an older adult will perform as well as an unpractised younger adult (Charness 1992). On intelligence tests, substantial practice effects counteract true declines of ageing and remain significant even with an interval of 7 years between tests.

Variability between individuals also increases as people age (Rabbit et al. 2004). Charness (1992) suggested that the critical issue in terms of age and performance is how the older person compensates for changes in processing speed and working memory. Obviously, the nature and amount of learning achieved in early and middle life impacts on the capacity of older adults when they are learning new skills and knowledge in later life in areas where they already have expertise. For example, Salthouse (1990) reported that architects preserved higher levels of spatial ability later in life than did non-architects (but maybe they always had superior spatial ability).

Why Do Older Adults Want to Learn?

Apart from the reasons described above, what motivates older adults to want to keep learning? Learning may be incidental, unanticipated or imposed. The large number of publications describing such events as the early stages of widowhood or the impact of becoming a carer, and the subsequent necessity of learning a range of unfamiliar tasks, present such examples. Alternatively, learning in later life may consist of the kind of individual reflection and life review that takes place in an unstructured and spasmodic way but which may lead to greater self-understanding and individual insight (Withnall 2000). The heterogeneity of the older population and the diversity of experience of different groups suggest that we need to find a way to understand the influence of different events and beliefs over the life course and to consider the effects of these on learning (Withnall 2000). Elders are also motivated to learn for self-fulfilment and pleasure. For example, Boulton-Lewis et al. (2006) found that the most frequent reasons given for wanting to keep learning were 'to keep the mind active, use the brain, exercise the mind, stay mentally stimulated, grow, attain goals, constantly learn, never stop'.

Motivation and confidence are critical to learning at any age, and particularly, so as people become older. Purdie and Boulton-Lewis (2001) found that the least important learning needs identified by older people were those associated with technology.

They stated that their most important learning needs were associated with transportation, health and safety. However, in earlier interview data in the same study, participants had suggested that the use of technology was something that they wanted to learn about; hence there was a difference between what they needed and what they wanted to learn. The strongest perceived barriers to learning were those associated with physical disabilities; the weakest barriers were those associated with interaction with other people. In general, participants were confident that they could successfully address learning needs related to health, safety, leisure and transportation but not those associated with technology. Boulton-Lewis et al. (2006) also found that although older adults learn more slowly, need more practice and their interests vary, in most cases their motivation is strong enough to learn new skills and to continue living fully through learning. Significant factors for continued active learning were being female, having good physical health, level of prior education, good mental/emotional health, being younger, living in regional areas, not being retired and being a higher income earner.

Negative attitudes held by others about older people learning need to be confronted. It should be generally acknowledged that older people are active and useful citizens who want to keep living their lives as fully as possible. As Stine-Morrow et al. (2007) stated the social construction of old age as a time when intellectual challenge is restricted (often implicitly and sometimes explicitly) encourages the very conditions that may not be favourable to cognitive and intellectual growth although opportunities for educational experiences in late life are becoming more available. Such ageist thinking needs to be addressed with sound arguments about older adults' desire and capability to keep on learning. If indeed learning keeps peoples' minds active, helps them in problem-solving and keeps them positively participating in life, then it makes them less dependent and actually saves governments money.

How Do Older People Want to Learn?

Older people vary in their preferences about how and where they want to learn. Some want organized courses and activities. Others want one-to-one tuition or to learn on their own. Some want formal courses and others want informal activities. A study by the Economic and Social Research Council (2003) in the UK found that many seniors prefer less formal forms of learning such as reading, conversation and watching educational television (2003). They also found that those who preferred formal learning were more likely to have had professional or semi-professional jobs, and the women were more likely to have worked.

Cruikshank (2003) asserted that one of the more significant ways in which people can be self-reinventive in ageing, particularly women, is through education but that educational system does not necessarily welcome older individuals. This situation could be overcome by allowing older people to audit courses in schools and universities and other institutions as they do in Elder Academies in Hong Kong (Labour and Welfare Bureau 2008). Lifelong learning is something of a catch phrase in education, and it is asserted that the basics of learning and knowledge laid down early in life are critical for learning as people age. This has implications for formal learning in schools, which should not only be a preparation for work but should also equip people with the skills and attitudes to keep on learning past their time in the workforce.

Some Opportunities for Learning and Education

Provisions for learning for older people vary from country to country. Some are within, or supported by, the formal system, and others are informal and rely on local initiatives. Some U3A groups in Australia and in the UK have been hosted by universities (chapter by Swindell), and others are local self-organized groups. There are programmes organized in universities in the UK that use university residences in holiday periods for courses for older people. Some universities in the USA that have built retirement accommodation on their campuses with the direct intention that the occupants can continue to learn by taking or auditing classes and Elderhostel programmes are popular internationally. Strathclyde University in Glasgow has a centre of excellence for the provision of lifelong learning for older people with more than 3,000 students each year participating in Senior Studies Institute (SSI) programmes. The SSI is unique in Scotland and has become internationally recognized for the quality of its educational programme (which focuses on lifelong learning, useful learning, widening access and research) and its expanding role in advising policy makers and business on age focused issues. It also promotes an intergenerational learning programme.

Some programmes have been initiated by older people themselves. Such programmes for older learners have proliferated in the USA in the last 20 years (Wolf 2009) and are generally of the non-formal type. A range of conditions has allowed this to occur including longer lives, improved health and economic status, better prior education, the popularity of lifelong learning theories that advance the benefits of learning and greater opportunities. However, as Swindell and Field warn in their chapters these initiatives are usually catering for more advantaged older people.

It has been asserted also that communities can promote engagement in various ways (Henkin and Zapf 2006). Communities can affect individuals in three ways: through settings and institutions in which they can participate, through norms and trust that grow from social networks and through systemic efforts that promote social cohesion and collective action. Hence, many groups have been formed in local communities to tap the potential for learning by the elderly. Toronto District School Board Senior's Daytime Program had about 1,200 enrolled in a range of programmes (2000–2006). The Elder Academy Scheme in Hong Kong (Labour and Welfare Bureau 2008) provides programmes that function in universities, primary and secondary schools and are supported by people of different generations. It is stated that they 'aim to encourage elders to continue learning, take care of their well being, have a sense of worthiness as well as to promote civic education, intergenerational solidarity and cross-sectoral collaboration'. The academies have management committees, and elders are represented on these. However, it is difficult to ascertain how the content of the learning programmes for these academies was determined.

Glanz and Neikrug (1997) reported positive outcomes from seniors themselves researching ageing which they claim was enriching, empowering and enabling. The Gerontology Institute at the University of Massachusetts, Boston has successfully encouraged groups of older people to become competent researchers (Caro 1999), and some University of the Third Age branches have also developed considerable expertise in training their members in the research process (Withnall 2000).

There are other activities, sometimes described as 'neurobics', which can be controlled by individuals themselves. *The Memory Bible* (Small 2003) contains mental strategies which claim to keep the brain'young' along with research-based advice on exercise, diet and lifestyle. There are similar books such as '*Keep your brain active*' (Katz and Rubin 1999), *20/20 Thinking* (Greenwood-Robinson 2003) that you can find on the Web as well as brain training programmes (such as the Nintendo version designed by Kawashima). There is not a great deal of empirical evidence to prove that these programmes work; however, intuitively, it would seem that they should. If physical exercise can help older people stay fit, then cognitive exercise should do the same for thought processes. The data supporting the aphorism that individuals should 'use it or lose it' are weak (Salthouse 2006) and mostly correlational. However, the study by Stine-Morrow et al. (2007) and the literature they review provide some support. They set up the Senior Odyssey, a team-based programme of creative problem-solving. They tested the engagement hypothesis in a field experiment and found that relative to controls, Senior Odyssey participants showed improved speed of processing, marginally improved divergent thinking and higher levels of mindfulness and need for cognition after the programme. Recent writing by Valenzuela (2009), as mentioned above, also considered neuroplasticity and neurogenesis.

Learning and Technology

Education provision for the elderly should include the use of technology; however, some people who are currently ageing have not had experience with computers and probably need (even if they do not want) to learn how to use them, for example, to access e-mail and information on the Web[4]. Such access, in theory, becomes more important if people have poor health and mobility. It allows them to obtain a wide range of services and information from home (Stadler and Teaster 2002). They can shop, bank, find out about health issues and entertainment and communicate with a wide range of others if they are computer literate.

[4] As Willis (2006) notes, this need might be a short-term phenomenon as elders in 10 years time will have had much more exposure to internet use.

Studies attest to the capacities and abilities of older people to learn how to use technology (Williamson et al. 1997; Scott 2001). A study of blocked and random practice schedules showed that older adults are capable of learning to use new technology (in this case a simulated ATM) through random practice even though they were slower, less accurate and more forgetful than younger users (Jamieson and Rogers 2000). In these kinds of contexts, one-on-one tuition for older users seems to offer increased potential for success. Older people have been encouraged to use ICT (Information Computer Technology) in specific settings such as computer clubs and libraries (Williamson et al. 1997). However, such opportunities are often in group situations and are not always easily acceptable or accessible by older people.

Models for the promotion of access to computer technology are being pioneered by entrepreneurs and communities in the USA (Morgan 2005). Computer company programmes and peer teaching (Grodsky and Gilbert 1998) are two such initiatives. Intergenerational learning has also been successful with children helping older people to master the necessary skills (Morgan 2005). Many seniors' organizations in Australia such as Australian Seniors Computer Clubs Association (ASCCA), Council on the Ageing (COTA), University of the Third Age (U3A) and SeniorNet actively promote computer tuition by older people for older people. The approaches focus particularly on complete beginners who may be fearful of the technology (Barker 2000).

A study of older adults in South England and Wales showed that, rather than resisting new computer technology, some older people's non-use was rather the perceived irrelevance of ICT in their lives, with 78% of non-users stating they had no need, and no interest, in using computers (Selwyn et al. 2003). This is probably the result of lack of earlier experience with the benefits of technology and presents a challenge in terms of convincing older adults that they can benefit from and be comfortable with it, in particular, those with low incomes, little relevant education or from ethnic minorities.

What Do Older People Want to Learn?

There is very little research that describes what older people themselves say they want and need to learn. There are statements about what others believe is necessary for them. Health professionals are concerned about how and why it is necessary to learn about health management (Kerschner and Pegues 1998; Crane 2001), and various studies suggest that health behaviour affects cognition in ageing. Others are concerned with elders learning about finance (Gregg 1993) and use of ICT (Stadler and Teaster 2002). Suggestions are made about the need to learn about technology if older people are to maintain their connections with its development and to take advantage of the benefits technology offers as described above.

Boulton-Lewis et al. (2005) found that older adults generally agreed that they needed and wanted to learn about things such as technology, new activities and leisure interests; however, respondents aged 50–64 were more likely to be interested, need and want to learn to keep up to date with new technology and make an effort to learn new thing and develop new talents, new skills and vocations, including aspects of technology.

Conclusion

There is limited empirical evidence, still mostly correlational, that education in early life or in ageing will halt the decline of cognitive powers. However, it will at least keep older people involved in enjoying and living life fully. It should assist with self-confidence and coping strategies, maintaining cognitive functioning and knowledge, health management, keeping up with technology developments, maintaining social relationships and encouraging wisdom. It may even improve neuroplasticity and support new neural pathways and utilize new brain cells.

Very little research has been undertaken where the elderly themselves are asked about learning and education. Withnall (2000) 'has suggested that a possible way forward in respect of the Third Age would be to change the current emphasis from *education* to *learning* and to investigate what meaning older people actually ascribe to learning by locating it within a life course perspective'. Elders themselves could be involved in the research. In obtaining empirical data, it has been argued that we need a new research paradigm that would place ageing itself at the centre of the debate and which incorporates older people themselves into the research process. In that way, it might be possible to move towards a new and more inclusive theory of lifelong learning that would have relevance for societies experiencing demographic and other kinds of change at an unprecedented rate. We need more data from older people themselves about their attitudes to learning and why, how and what they want to learn. It would also be valuable to have more data about whether such learning has measurable positive benefits.

References

Ardelt, M. (2000). Intellectual versus wisdom-related knowledge: The case for a different kind of learning in the later years of life. *Educational Gerontology, 26*, 771–789.

Arsenault, N., & Anderson, G. (1998). New learning horizons for older adults. *Journal of Physical Education, Recreation and Dance, 69*(3), 27–31.

Australian Government Productivity Commission. (2005). *Economic implications of an ageing Australia* (Research Report). Canberra: Australian Government Productivity Commission.

Barker, N. (2000). *Computing for the mortally terrified and other fantastic futures.* Paper presented at the 2000 Fulbright symposium: Implications for an Ageing Population, Perth, Western Australia.

Boulton-Lewis, G. (1997). Information processing, memory, age and adult learning. In P. Sutherland (Ed.), *Adult learning: A reader*. London: Kogan Page.

Boulton-Lewis, G. M., Buys, L., Lovie-Kitchin, J., Courtney, M., Edwards, H., Anderson, D., Nayak, R., & Zlobicki, M. T. (2005, August). *Learning and active ageing*. Paper presented at the EARLI Conference, August 23–27, 2005, Nicosia, Cyprus.

Boulton-Lewis, G. M., Buys, L., & Lovie-Kitchin, J. (2006). Learning and active aging. *Educational Gerontology, 32*(4), 271–282.

Bowling, A., & Iliffe, S. (2006). Which model of successful ageing should be used? Baseline findings from a British longitudinal survey of ageing. *Age and Ageing, 35*(6), 607–614.

Butler, R. N. (2002). The study of productive aging. *Journals of Gerontology, Series B: Psychological Sciences and Social Sciences, 57*(6), S323.

Caro, F. (1999). *Training for older people in applied social research methods*. Boston: University of Massachusetts Press.

Charness, N. (1992). Age and expertise: Responding to Talland's challenge. In I. W. Poon, D. C. Rubin, & B. A. Wilson (Eds.), *Everyday cognition in adulthood and later life*. Cambridge: Cambridge University Press.

Crane, P. B. (2001). I want to know: Exploring how older women acquire health knowledge after myocardial infarction. *Journal of Women & Aging, 13*(4), 3.

Cruikshank, M. (2003). *Learning to be old: Gender, culture and aging*. Lanham: Littlefield Publishers.

Dench, S., & Regan, J. (2000). *Learning in later life: Motivation and impact*. Nottingham: DfEE.

Department for Community Development, Government of Western Australia. (2006). *Western Australia's seniors active ageing benchmark indicators: An initiative of generations together – The Western Australian active ageing strategy*. Retrieved March 4, 2008, from http://www.community.wa.gov.au/DFC/Communities/Seniors/Publications/Active_Ageing_Benchmark_Indicators.htm

Economic and Social Research Council. (2003). Swindon, UK: Polaris House. Retrieved January 13, 2010, from http://www.esrc.ac.uk

Glanz, D., & Neikrug, S. (1997). Seniors as researchers in the study of aging: Learning and doing. *The Gerontologist, 37*(6), 823–826.

Greenwood-Robinson, M. (2003). *20/20 thinking*. New York: Avery Trade.

Gregg, D. W. (1993). Financial gerontology. *Journal of the American Society of CLU and ChFC, 47*(2), 32. Retrieved from the ABI/INFORM Global database (Document ID: 284197).

Grodsky, T., & Gilbert, G. C. (1998). Seniors travel the information superhighway. *Parks and Recreation Arlington, 33*(6), 70–74.

Henkin, N., & Zapf, J. (2006). How communities can promote civic engagement of people age 50-plus. *Generations, 30*(4), 72–77.

Government Logistics Department. *Hong Kong Population Projections 2010–2039*. Hong Kong: Government Logistics Department.

Horn, J. L., & Hofer, S. M. (1992). Major abilities and development in the adult period. In R. J. Sternberg & C. A. Berg (Eds.), *Intellectual development*. Cambridge/New York: Cambridge University Press.

Jamieson, B. A., & Rogers, W. A. (2000). Age-related effects of blocked and random practice schedules on learning a new technology. *Journals of Gerontology, Series B: Psychological Sciences and Social Sciences, 55B*(6), 343–353.

Katz, I. C., & Rubin, M. (1999). *Keep your brain active: 83 neurobic exercises to help prevent memory loss and increase mental fitness*. New York: Workman Publishing.

Kerschner, H., & Pegues, J. M. (1998). Productive aging: A quality of life agenda. *Journal of the American Dietetic Association, 98*(12), 1445–1448.

Kirasic, K. C., Allen, G. L., Dobson, S. H., Shannon, H., & Binder, K. S. (1996). Aging, cognitive resources and declarative learning. *Psychology and Aging, 11*(4), 658–670.

Kotulak, R. (1997). *Inside the brain: Revolutionary discoveries of how the mind works*. Kansas City: Andrews Michael Publishing.

Labour and Welfare Bureau. (2008). *The Government of the Hong Kong Special Administrative Region, Government and elderly commission to expand elder academy scheme*, Press release, June 13, 2008. Retrieved January 21, 2008, from http://www.lwb.gov.hk/eng/press/13062008htm.S

Marton, F. (1988). *Phenomenography: Exploring different conceptions of reality*. New York: Praeger.

Morgan, R. E. (2005). Technology greets the age wave. *The Gerontologist, 45*(5), 704–710.

National Seniors Productive Ageing Centre. (2005). Active and productive ageing: What is the real experience of Australians? *Research Bulletin, 1*(1).

Phelan, E. A., Anderson, L. A., LaCroix, A. Z., & Larson, E. B. (2004). Older adults' views of successful aging – How do they compare with researchers' definitions? *Journal of the American Geriatrics Society, 52*(2), 211–216.

Purdie, N., & Boulton-Lewis, G. (2001). The learning needs of older adults. *Educational Gerontology, 29*, 129–149.

Rabbit, D., Diggle, P., Holland, F., & McInnes, L. (2004). Practice and drop-out effects during a 17-year longitudinal study of cognitive aging. *Journals of Gerontology, Series B: Psychological Sciences and Social Sciences, 59*(2), 84–97.

Salthouse, T. A. (1985). *A theory of cognitive aging*. New York: Elsevier.

Salthouse, T. A. (1990). Cognitive competence and expertise in ageing. In J. E. Birren & K. W. Schaie (Eds.), *Handbook of the psychology of aging* (3rd ed., pp. 310–319). San Diego: Academic.

Salthouse, T. A. (2006). Mental exercise and mental aging: Evaluating the validity of the "use it or lose it" hypothesis. *Perspectives on Psychological Science, 1*, 68–87.

Scott, H. (2001). Old dogs learning new clicks – Older Americans in the information age. *Council on the Ageing, 12*. Retrieved January 13, 2009, from http://cotaover50s.org/an/acota/cota.Aust/ecommerc.htm

Selwyn, N., Gorard, S., Furlong, J., & Madden, L. (2003). Older adults' use of information and communication technology in everyday life. *Ageing & Society, 23*, 561–582.

Senior Studies Institute, University of Strathclyde, Glasgow. (n.d.). Retrieved January 13, 2010, http://www.strath.ac.uk/cll/seniorstudiesinstitute/

Small, G. (2003). *The memory bible: An innovative strategy for keeping your brain young*. New York: Hyperion.

Smits, C. H., Deeg, D. M., & Schmand, B. (1999). Cognitive functioning and health as determinants of mortality in older populations. *American Journal of Epidemiology, 150*(9), 978–986.

Stadler, K. M., & Teaster, P. B. (2002). Aging, nutrition, technology, web sites, older people. *Journal of Nutrition Education and Behavior: Nutrition Education and Older Adults, 34*, S67–S68.

Stine-Morrow, E. A. L., Parisi, J. M., Morrow, D. G., Greene, J., & Park, D. C. (2007). An engagement model of cognitive optimization through adulthood. *Journals of Gerontology: Series B Psychological Sciences and Social Sciences Special Issue 1: Cognitive Interventions and Aging, 62B*, 62–69.

Summer, A. (2007). The silver tsunami: One educational strategy for preparing to meet America's next wave of underserved. *Journal of Health Care for the Poor and Underserved, 18*(3), 503–509.

Toronto District School Board. (2000–2006). *The learn 4 life brochure: General interest courses for adults, seniors' daytime courses*. Toronto: Toronto Continuing Education Office. Toronto District School Board.

United Nations Department of Economic and Social Affairs, Population Division. (2007). *World Population aging 2007*. New York: United Nations.

Valenzuela, M. J. (2009). *It's never too late to change your mind*. Sydney, Australia: ABC Books.

Van Dijk, K. R. A., Van Gerven, P. W. M., Van Boxtel, M. P. J., Van der Elst, W., & Jolles, J. (2008). No protective effects of education during normal cognitive aging. Results from the 6-year follow-up of the Maastricht aging study. *Psychology and Aging, 23*(1), 119–130.

Williamson, K., Bow, A., & Wale, K. (1997). Encouraging public Internet use by older people: A comparative study of city and rural area. *Rural Society, 7*(3/4), 3–11.

Willis, S. L. (2006). Technology and learning in current and future generations of elders. *Generations, 30*(2), 44–46.

Willis, S. L., & Schaie, K. W. (2006). A coconstructionist view of the third age: The case of cognition. *Annual Review of Gerontology and Geriatrics, 26*, 131–151.

Withnall, A. (2000). *Older learners – Issues and perspectives* (Working papers of the Global colloquium on supporting lifelong learning) [online]. Milton Keynes: Open University. Retrieved March 14, 2002, from http//www.open.ac.uk/lifelong-learning

Wolf, M. A. (2009). Older adulthood. In P. Jarvis (Ed.), *The Routledge international handbook of lifelong learning*. London: Routledge.

World Health Organization (WHO). (2002). *Active ageing: A policy framework.* Retrieved April 18, 2005, from http://www.who.int/hpr/ageing/ActiveAgeingPolicyFrame.pdf

Chapter 4
Successful Ageing and International Approaches to Later-Life Learning

Rick Swindell

Introduction

A combination of low mortality and low fertility will continue to have a marked impact on the population of many countries for decades to come. By 2050, older people will outnumber children in most parts of the world, with the exception of Africa. In some countries, for example Italy, Portugal, Greece and Spain, older people will outnumber children by as much as four to one (The Research Council of Norway 2010).

Scientific, technological, educational and other social advances continue to increase the average life expectancy in most countries and those in the oldest age range now comprise the fastest growing sector in the total population. For example, in developed countries, the fastest growing population sector is aged 85 years and older.

However, population ageing is viewed by some as something of a two-edged sword. Population ageing is undoubtedly the confirmation of a society's coming of age; the reward for vast investments over many decades to the reforms and developments that created the conditions for most of its citizens to reasonably expect to live to a ripe old age. Lives are now saved that previously would have been lost. The other edge of the population-ageing sword is associated with rapidly increasing costs (Productivity Commission 2010). Disability rises with age, and longevity also brings increasing costs associated with complex chronic care for age-related diseases such as dementia and diabetes as well as geriatric and palliative care.

Technology would appear to have an important role to play in helping to maintain the quality of life of society's most vulnerable people. For example, technology has the potential to transform aged care and healthcare. Smart houses equipped with

R. Swindell (✉)
U3AOnline at Griffith University, Brisbane, QLD, Australia
e-mail: ricks1912@gmail.com

G.M. Boulton-Lewis and M. Tam (eds.), *Active Ageing, Active Learning: Issues and Challenges*, Education in the Asia-Pacific Region: Issues, Concerns and Prospects 15,
DOI 10.1007/978-94-007-2111-1_4,

intelligent devices that enable independent living, social participation and better and less costly access to medical services and care are being tested in many countries (Soar et al. 2011). Regardless of technological advances, however, it seems highly likely that the sheer number of people entering their Fourth Age will cause costs to continue to rise rapidly. (The Fourth Age is the final stage of life, during which frail elderly people require considerable daily support. Many people in their Fourth Age retain sound mental function but within a failing body.)

Lifelong learning also has an important role to play in an ageing society. Renewed interest in the benefits of lifelong learning is shaping new thinking right across the lifelong learning continuum. In the UK, the Inquiry into the Future of Lifelong Learning (IFLL) brought together experts from government, business, academia, trade unions, public service, providers, the voluntary and community sector, as well as learners, in a process to identify a broad consensus for the future for lifelong learning. The 2 year inquiry sought: to articulate a broad rationale for public and private investment in lifelong learning, reappraisal of the social and cultural value attached to lifelong learning by policy makers and the public, and development of new perspectives on policy and practice. Recommendations are wide-ranging and cover four main learning entitlements – digital, health, finances and civic responsibilities. Four new lifelong learning population groups that account for new demographic clusters are proposed – up to 25, 25–50, 50–75 and 75 and older. Schuller and Watson (n.d.) summarize the new thinking that has evolved from the IFLL inquiry. For every £55 spent on learning in the UK £47 goes to the 18–24 group, £6 to the 25–29 group, £1 to the 50–74 group, and 29p to the 75+ group. The ideas propose dramatic departures from historical norms.

Lifelong learning advocates argue that a much fairer allocation of funding is now needed in recognition of changing demographics and a growing understanding that learning in later life can help older people to stay active, engaged with society and healthy. The transformative benefits of later-life learning programmes suggest creative and comparatively inexpensive ways for assisting older people to take part in the kinds of activity which give them the best chances for maximizing their independence in later life. McNair (2009) calls for the introduction of many more and better learning opportunities for the rapidly growing Fourth Age population in the UK, enabling them to maintain identity, health, social engagement and well-being during the final stages of life.

The European Commission is addressing population ageing on a number of fronts and the benefits of lifelong learning feature prominently. LARA (Learning A Response to Ageing) is an action response to an ageing population funded by the European Commission. The LARA project has developed a suite of training and self-study programmes for teachers and managers of adult education to develop and deliver learning that is responsive to the demands and opportunities of ageing (LARA n.d.).

An emerging body of evidence suggests there are important health benefits which are associated with lifelong learning. Harper (2008) notes that mental development, brain capacity and longevity are closely associated. As the relationship between mental capacity and physical health becomes clearer, education will form a growing element of personal enhancement. She further notes that the UK government policy has tended to think of demographic ageing as leading to large numbers of old people, rather than large numbers of people who are simply living longer – many of them with increasingly active healthy lives (Harper 2008, p. 10). A compelling recent summation of the potential contribution that lifelong learning can make to a wider society comes from The Foresight Project on Mental Capital and Wellbeing (Beddington et al. 2008). The project took a whole-of-life approach in reaching its conclusion that countries must learn how to capitalize on their citizens' cognitive resources if they are to prosper. More than 450 experts and stakeholders from 16 countries were involved in the review of state-of-the-art scientific and other evidence to investigate the challenges and opportunities that lie ahead in the next 20 years. The recommendations regarding older learners were particularly noteworthy. The study recommended that 'as people move into older age, learning should be encouraged and actively promoted, as this can protect against cognitive decline' (p. 1058).

Successful Ageing

Refocusing ageing policy away from expensive remedial actions and towards low-cost, preventative interventions that empower older people and keeps them independent and participating in their communities for as long as possible is a feature of many forward-planning ageing-strategy documents. What is it that keeps some people aged in their 80s, 90s and older, who continue to age successfully, engaging optimistically and independently with everyday life, while others who are many years younger may have already lost their independence?

During the past few decades a growing interest in the science of ageing has resulted in large, well-funded, multidisciplinary studies which continue to provide new evidence-based answers to the processes of ageing. Successful ageing, ageing well, healthy ageing, productive ageing and positive ageing are among the evidence-based ageing models that have evolved from large studies. The models differ from each other in emphasis rather than absolute content (Friedrich 2003). However, all models focus on only a small number of choices that individuals must follow if they want to maximize their chances of retaining their independence and minimize the costs associated with frail and dependent ageing.

The MacArthur Foundation Study of Successful Ageing (Rowe and Kahn 1999) illustrates the substantial gains in understanding of ageing that can flow from a large, interdisciplinary research study. The study, which was actually a coherent set of dozens of individual research projects led by 16 leading researchers in the USA, drawn from across the broad spectrum of gerontology, including biology, neuroscience, neuropsychology, epidemiology, sociology, genetics, psychology, neurology, physiology and geriatric medicine, was the most extensive and comprehensive multidisciplinary study on ageing in America. The Successful Ageing model, which was an outcome of the collective findings, outlines three fundamental attributes of a successfully ageing individual. These are:

- Low risk of disease and disease-related disability
- High mental and physical function
- Active engagement with life by maintaining social networks and continuing to do interesting things

Each of these three major components of the model is important in itself although they are interrelated. They also may be somewhat hierarchical in that the absence of disease and disability may make it easier to maintain mental and physical function, and this in turn may enable, but not guarantee, engagement with life.

There are five lifestyle choices which are associated with the three major attributes of the Rowe and Kahn Successful Ageing model, and each of these will now briefly be discussed.

Low Risk of Disease and Disease-Related Disability

Many people consider that the risk of disease is entirely down to the lottery of genetics; did we choose our parents wisely? The role of genetics in successful ageing is undoubtedly important but the influence appears to have been overstated. Family studies, population studies, adoption studies and studies of twins, which were all components of the MacArthur Study, allowed the interplay between nature and nurture to be separated. For all but the most strongly determined genetic diseases, environment and lifestyle have a powerful impact on the likelihood of actually developing the disorder (Rowe and Kahn 1999). Thus, decisions to exercise regularly; cut out smoking; eat less salt, fat and red meat; eat more fruit, vegetables and fish; reduce alcohol intake; lose weight, and avoid over exposure to sunlight are just some of the well-publicized environmental and lifestyle choices that we can adopt to directly lower the risk of future disease and disability.

But what happens if, despite all our precautions, life-threatening disease strikes? It seems that even after health problems occur, older people can successfully continue to engage with life if they adopt health control strategies like seeking help, staying on prescribed medicines, devoting time and energy to address the challenges, and being committed to overcoming threats to physical health. For example, in a 2-year follow-up study, Wrosch and Schulz (2008) found that elderly participants who were proactive and persistent in countering health problems showed greater physical and mental health benefits than those who were not. Their findings suggest that once disease strikes, active control strategies play an important role in the maintenance of older adults' physical health.

High Mental and Physical Function

Mental Function

For the many older adults who regularly engage in learning activities, maintaining high cognitive function would probably be the highest priority among the elements of the Successful Ageing model. After all, if the brain is no longer functioning effectively, could or would an individual continue to carry out the other elements of the model?

Memory and learning can be maintained or revitalized even quite late in life. Rowe and Kahn (1999) reported on one study in which the lives of more than 1,000 high-functioning older people were followed for 8 years to determine the factors that might predict successful physical and mental ageing. Many reported that they sustain their mental ability as they age by actively working at keeping their minds sharp. The research suggests that 'this is part of a cycle that promotes mental ability: the more you have, the more you do; the more you do, the more you preserve' (p. 130). Education was found to be the strongest predictor of sustained mental function in later life. The authors speculated on two possible effects that could explain this link. First, education in early life may have a direct beneficial effect on brain circuitry; or second, education may set a lifelong pattern (e.g. reading, chess, Mahjong, bridge, crossword puzzles) that serves to maintain cognitive function in old age. Furthermore, some actions to avert or minimize cognitive loss can be undertaken at any age. With training 'elderly men and women who have experienced some cognitive decline can…offset approximately two decades of memory loss' (p. 137).

The importance of making good lifestyle choices was similarly revealed by Vaillant (2002) who followed the lifestyles of groups of men and women from adolescence until age 80 to deduce the attributes of those who were seen to be the most successful agers. His study, which ran for 60 years, suggested that successful ageing from age 70–80 could be predicted by variables assessed before age 50. The importance of intellectual curiosity and lifelong learning is one of the choices of people who age successfully.

Maintaining High Physical Function

The benefits of exercise have been known for many years. Numerous studies continue to show that exercise reduces the risk of cardiovascular disease and overall mortality risk, as well as promoting psychological well-being. A regular combination of stretching, strengthening, balance and cardio-vascular exercises appears to have wide-ranging physiological benefits including, perhaps somewhat surprisingly, promoting cognitive function. (See for example, Erickson et al. 2010; Lautenschlager et al. 2008; Smith et al. 2011).

Exactly why exercise has a positive effect on brain function is not yet known. One suggestion is that exercise helps to maintain the health of blood vessels in the brain, helping to ensure a steady supply of oxygen and nutrients to areas of the brain that are critical for thinking and memory. Physical activity may also stimulate the release of factors critical for brain cell growth, increasing resistance to damage caused by dementia. Andel et al. (2008) studied exercise patterns in 50-year olds and followed up 30 years later. They found that exercise at midlife reduces the odds of dementia in older adulthood, and concluded that exercise interventions should be explored as a potential strategy for delaying disease onset. Erikson et al. (2011), in a randomized controlled study showed that a programme of aerobic exercise over the course of a year can increase the size of the hippocampus in adults aged 55–80. The hippocampus is part of the brain that is the key to memory and spatial navigation, which shrinks in late adulthood leading to impaired memory and increased risk for dementia. They conclude that their findings clearly indicate that aerobic exercise is neuroprotective and that starting an exercise regimen later in life is not futile for either enhancing cognition or augmenting brain volume (p. 5).

Active Engagement with Life

The Rowe and Kahn (1999) Successful Ageing model involves two separate elements to active engagement with life, namely maintaining close social networks and doing interesting things.

Maintaining Social Networks

It's an unfortunate fact of life that the closer we are to the wrong end of the lifelong learning continuum, the greater the chances are of losing important social networks and becoming socially isolated. The most devastating of the risk factors is, of course, death of a very close friend. However there are many other risks to social networks, including divorce, retiring to a new location, giving up driving, prolonged bouts of ill health or incapacity, and caring for a sick friend or spouse. The impact of these and similar unexpected calamitous events on older persons' social networks is readily apparent from demographic data that are routinely available in many countries.

Without special friends we run the risk of entering a downward spiral of depression, leading to further ill health, leading to greater depression and perhaps the danger of loss of independence or, in the extreme, suicide. Indeed, the importance of social networks is one of the most robust of findings from social science research (Bowling 1994). Study after study shows that a small group of special friends is essential to well-being throughout life. The special friends are those we turn to for advice and support to get us through those low periods when the going gets tough. Social networks are so strongly linked to health and general well-being that a paper published as long ago as 1988 in the journal *Science* equated the health risks caused by fragmentation of social networks with those associated with the early years of smoking (House et al. 1988). More recent findings continue to refine the specific benefits of social networks. For example, a nationally representative study of Ertel et al. (2008) provided evidence that social integration delays memory loss among elderly Americans.

In the rush of everyday life, the world seems to be becoming an increasingly lonely place, and social networks have become harder to retain or renew (Dorling et al. 2008). Neighbours come and go without engaging with their communities; the pressure of working-life keeps growing; jobs keep changing; individuals feel they have less of a voice in society; new demands are placed on members of society to keep up with technological 'innovations', and so on. For many participants in later-life learning organizations, developing new social networks with like-minded colleagues is an important feature of their membership.

Doing Interesting Things

The second element of actively engaging with life is doing interesting things. Of course, the domain of 'interesting things' is subjective and open-ended. In other words, what is interesting for one older person may hold no attraction at all for another. Consequently, attributing a specific health and well-being outcome to a particular 'engaging' activity requires targeted research. Volunteering is a popular example of an interesting activity for many older people, and volunteering continues to be widely studied. It seems that everyone can be a winner from voluntarism; participants, recipients of the services and the wider economy alike. For the volunteers themselves, it seems that those who regularly engage in their voluntary activities enjoy better health and live longer, thanks to the stimulating environments and sense of purpose engendered by their activities. Zedlewski and Butrica (2007) summarized the outcomes of ten studies published since 1999 which documented the significant positive associations between volunteer activity and decreased mortality and depression, improved health and strength, greater happiness and enhanced cognitive ability. Barron et al. (2009) studied volunteering among older adults in fair health and concluded that productive activity such as volunteering may be an effective community-based approach to health promotion for older adults. It seems that volunteers are helping themselves while helping the wider community.

The Rowe and Kahn (1999) model of successful ageing involves personal choices that relate directly to physical and mental health, as well as wider psychosocial considerations that deal with the 'whole' person. Nevertheless, their approach has been criticized for being overly narrow and too focused on measurable health outcomes rather than including intangible aspects that are important to older people themselves. For example, many older people who are satisfied with life in general, rate their subjective health highly even though they may have severe health problems of a kind which would earn them a 'poor health' rating from a narrow medical focus on disease or disability. In addition, Glass (2003) argues that a more complete successful ageing model must include recognition of existential aspects of life which are important to many older people, such as spirituality (not merely in the narrow doctrinal sense). Despite this criticism however, the five elements which make up the three components of the successful ageing model, namely:

Low risk of disease and disease-related disability
Maintaining high mental function
Maintaining high physical function
Maintaining strong social networks
Doing interesting things

Provide a convenient, evidence-based checklist which can help older people to monitor their lifestyle choices.

Successful Ageing and Later-Life Learning

An almost inevitable outcome of more people living longer and placing increasing demands on social service budgets is that individuals will be required to fund more of the costs associated with their own aged care. In the introduction to this chapter, a growing interest in the important role that lifelong learning will play in population ageing is discussed. New ageing policy action is needed to more fairly balance resource allocations and better account for the major changes in demography that are rapidly taking place.

A growing body of evidence underpins the elements of the successful ageing model. The model suggests strategies which people of all ages can engage in to maximize their chances for independence and, implicitly, minimize the costs to be paid for their future aged care. Three of the five successful ageing elements, namely cognitively challenging activity, doing interesting things and developing new social networks are fundamental attributes of most lifelong learning programmes. The other two elements – keeping the body active through exercise, and learning about the kinds of lifestyle choices that minimize the chances of disease and disability – could be seamlessly interwoven into a new lifelong learning curriculum for all ages and particularly in an increased emphasis on later life learning where their benefits seem clear. Indeed, an important health benefit associated with later-life learning is singled out in The Foresight Project (Beddington et al. 2008), which advocates society's need to encourage and actively promote learning in older age as this can protect against cognitive decline (p. 1058).

A key message here is *active* promotion of learning in later life. By and large, the latter end of the lifelong learning spectrum in many countries has received little more than lip service from governments and their allied ageing policies. Any active support for later-life learning opportunities has tended to focus on upgrading older workers' skills so that they can continue in, or return to the paid workforce. Schuller and Watson (n.d.) list a number of characteristics of people in the UK who are under represented in lifelong learning activities. They are people who have less money, do not have a paid job, are older, and are disabled. For many in the older population all those characteristics apply. Governments will need to substantially reallocate resources in order to encourage older people to take part in later-life learning activities in much greater numbers than they do at present.

Some Later-Life Learning Organizations and Successful Ageing

The appendix to this chapter describes a number of major later-life learning organizations that are popular in various countries. One of the defining characteristics of many of these organizations is that they are driven by grassroots member volunteers, and many of them have little or no need for substantial external funding or paid teaching or administrative staff. In other words, older people themselves have voted with their feet. They have chosen to become involved in later-life learning, generally in the absence of guiding policy direction from governments. Experts of all kinds retire and these older, expert volunteers provide the foundation for the success of these organizations. As discussed earlier, volunteering has many benefits, including the improved health and well-being of volunteers themselves.

One of the best known of these volunteer-driven, later-life learning organizations is the U3A (University of the Third Age) or UTA, as it is called in many countries. As shown in the appendix, there are many variations of this approach worldwide, and most provide activities that encompass four or all five successful ageing elements (Rowe and Kahn 1999). Some approaches such as the Lifelong Learning Institutes (LLI) in North America, or the French UTA model, which is popular in many countries, are based at universities or colleges where members have access to high-level learning and teaching resources, such as libraries and computers. However, the teaching and programme administration is mainly or solely carried out by skilled retirees, and the formal university system has little or no say over the educational content and process. By contrast, the self-help U3A approach, which is also popular in many countries, is based entirely within the community. Courses and activities are often run from convenient venues such as free or subsidized community halls, local government community rooms and even members' homes. In China, the Universities for the Aged use a combination of revered older teachers who are paid a stipend, and older and young unpaid volunteers, to teach a curriculum which covers compulsory subjects like health and exercise, as well as a wide range of academic and leisure courses. In other countries, different combinations of second- and third-age expertise provide popular programmes for older people that encompass most of or all five elements of Rowe and Kahn's (1999) successful ageing model. Some of the programmes feature courses related to lifestyle choices that lower the risk of disease and disability; all provide intellectually challenging activities; most provide fitness-related activities that encourage participants to take up new exercise programmes in the company of like-minded individuals; all are run in social environments; and all involve doing things that participants are interested in.

Older People and Novel Communications Technologies

Frequently, older people become isolated from their mainstream communities by a daunting array of constraints that make it difficult for them to continue to engage with life. Even in large, well-resourced cities which offer many opportunities for older people to do interesting things, abrupt changes to circumstance such as illness, incapacity or being thrust into the role of caregiver, leave many older people with few compensatory options to choose from. Isolation is a threat to individuals' abilities to take part in successful ageing activities within their immediate communities.

Communications technologies have considerable potential for motivating isolated older people to engage with life in entirely new ways. In the early 1990s, a series of studies was undertaken to investigate the possibility of setting up a virtual U3A for frail elderly people with sound minds. The studies showed that older volunteer teachers and learners alike were not averse to using novel technology to learn new things (Swindell et al. 1994, 1992). In one of the studies, three groups, each of six frail elderly people aged from 58 to 92 years old, who were confined to their homes by illness or incapacity, showed measurable improvements in their quality of life over the course of an 8-week educational programme delivered via teleconference. The programmes were taught by volunteer U3A tutors who were trained in the techniques of teleconferencing. A trained nurse interacted with the participants throughout the study to monitor basic health data and record observations. The well-being of participants improved over the course of the study and several developed new social networks as a result of interacting with like-minded others within their virtual groups. They stated that the educational programme was the catalyst that induced them to experiment with a novel method of communicating and exploring beyond their physically and socially constrained horizons (Swindell and Mayhew 1996).

The isolated participants in the above studies were connected by telephone; therefore, the location of the U3A tutors was irrelevant. The Internet would clearly have been a more flexible and cost-effective medium than teleconferencing for carrying out the above virtual U3A trials. However, in the 1990s, computers and the Internet were unknown quantities for most retirees. The situation is quite different today. Although a large disparity still exists between the numbers of older and younger Internet users, growing numbers of older people are happy to come to grips with technology that played little or no part in their earlier lives. For example, Madden (2010) reported on the rapid adoption of social media by older adults in the USA. In 2009–2010, social networking use among Internet users aged 50 and older nearly doubled from 22% to 42%; for those aged 65 and older, usage doubled from 13% to 26%. In the same period, social network uptake by the 18–29 age range grew from 76% to 86%. The importance of the Internet as a medium for improving social networks among older North Americans is further reinforced by Rainee et al. (2011) who show that email is the primary way that older Internet users maintain contact with friends, families and colleagues.

The potential of the Internet seems limitless for opening up new learning opportunities and increased prospects for virtual social connectedness. The implications for older people are particularly exciting. Once they have learnt the comparatively trivial skill of using the Internet, and provided they have easily accessible and inexpensive access to the Internet, a new world of successful ageing resources is at their fingertips. Supportive information from governments, NGOs, leisure organizations and other agencies is expensive to provide in conventional print form and increasingly accessible only through the Internet. Online shopping and banking removes another stress for disabled, ill and other isolated older people. Free Web 2.0 applications, such as wikis, Skype and social networking sites, have considerable scope for widening the range of socially and intellectually enriching activities in the daily lives of older people, allowing them to communicate with family and like-minded others when and if they want to. However, using the Internet may also have previously unrecognized direct health benefits for older 'surfers'. The process of decision making via the Internet may also help to exercise and improve brain function. Research with older people who surf the Internet shows that the process triggers key centres in the brain involved in decision making and complex reasoning when they make decisions about what to click on in order to pursue more information. This research, which studied brain activity in real time, showed that Internet searching engages a much greater extent of neural circuitry than reading does (Small et al. 2009).

International Cooperation and the Internet

Cooperation among older learners is not a novel idea. As outlined in the appendix to this chapter, large learning networks such as IAUTA, the Third Age Trust in the UK, and the EIN in North America have been in existence for several decades. These networks would never have started if older learners had not been prepared to share. However, the Internet has dramatically increased the possibilities for low-cost international cooperation between later-life learning organizations. Cost, national borders, language, race or creed need no longer serve as barriers to lifelong learners of good will who want to share with other like-minded people anywhere.

This section discusses two examples of international projects in which volunteers work cooperatively via the Internet in successful ageing projects carried out for the benefit of an international community of older learners.

U3A Online

The first international virtual U3A, U3A Online, was set up in 1998 in recognition of the fact that many people, both old and young, are socially isolated. Via the Internet, they can engage with other like-minded people around the world in intellectually and socially stimulating virtual activities, including volunteering.

From the outset the project has had a global focus. The initial Project Reference Group comprised U3A enthusiasts from Australia, New Zealand and the UK who recognized the potential of the Internet for harnessing the expertise of a worldwide cadre of volunteers who would provide low-cost, intellectually stimulating courses and resources for a world community of learners and other volunteers.

As with any self-help U3A, all the administration and teaching in U3A Online is carried out by volunteers. No one is paid. Governance and administration occurs through regular virtual meetings. Discussion and voting takes place by electronic forum, email and Skype. Annual general meetings, at which office bearers are elected by members, are held online. At various times volunteers on the management team have been elected from Australia, New Zealand, the UK and Poland. It is commonplace for the majority of volunteers to work closely together for many years, but never physically meet.

An all volunteer-based virtual learning–teaching organization has few expensive overheads. There are no salaries to pay, no premises to maintain, no expensive insurance costs and no health and safety constraints. In addition, since 2002, Griffith University in Brisbane, Australia has hosted the entire operation free of charge on university servers, as part of its service to the wider community. Courses are delivered via the University online course delivery platform, also free of charge. The net result is that fees are kept extremely low. For example, in 2011, the annual U3A Online membership fee was A$25. (For comparison a movie ticket costs about A$13.) Membership is open to all older people from any country, and to younger people with disabilities. At the time of writing this chapter in early 2011, 39 courses were available to U3A Online members with others in various stages of completion, all written, edited and taught by volunteers. All courses are free to members for self study and are available 365 days a year. For an additional fee, a further 13 courses are available to members through a cooperative arrangement with the Third Age Trust in the UK, which has provided online courses for its UK members since 2000. Courses are equivalent to 8 or 9 weeks of work. Depending on the availability of volunteer tutors, members may opt to pay an additional A$5 to join tutor-led options, during which participants interact with the leader and with others in the course by online forum and email. Participants and tutors live in any country so live interaction, for example, by Skype, is generally impracticable.

The concept has clearly made a difference to the health and quality of life of many isolated older people. For example:

> I'll go as far as to say that being totally absorbed in my most recent online course has saved my sanity this year.

> I am partially blind with limited short sight. I am extremely grateful to U3A as I now have an interest at home – am happy working on my own and life has again a meaning.

> I care for my wife who has Alzheimer's. Have done so for the last 8 years.

Further comments and a description of all courses can be found on www.u3aonline.org.au.

Site licences are an additional service available to any U3A-style organization in any country, and these can be purchased from U3A Online for A$20 per course per year.

A site licence permits organizations to print unlimited copies of any one of the U3A Online courses in any year, and these notes may be given free of charge to members of the organization for face-to-face teaching. In addition, any new U3A-style organization in any country qualifies for one free site licence to help them get started. The course notes have all been written and illustrated by expert volunteers in their fields, and, in some cases, these run to more than 100 pages when printed.

All courses and resources are in English. U3A Online is now working with an organization that is dedicated to providing online services for CALD (Culturally and linguistically diverse) people. The intention is for U3A Online courses and resources to be provided in many languages and to provide CALD members with new volunteering opportunities, and virtual social networks and learning communities with native speakers elsewhere.

A monthly email newsletter called GEMs is freely available to anyone in any country. GEMs contains links to free Internet courses and services; links to summaries of the latest scientific research about successful ageing topics; and technology hints and ideas.

U3A Online and Constituency Research

The fundamental strength of the constituency research approach is that it entails research 'with' rather than research 'on' older people. The difference between 'with' and 'on' may not matter too much in large-scale tick-a-box surveys. However, if much richer findings are needed, these are more likely to arise from interviews carried out by peers who are perceived to have primary empathy with the participants, rather than by younger researchers whose appearance, manner of dress, language, general persona and time constraints may create barriers to in-depth communication.

U3A Online has sponsored a number of research/development studies that have been carried out in association with member researchers and published in peer-reviewed literature. 'A voice worth listening to' is an example of a novel constituency research project undertaken exclusively by third agers (Braxton et al. 2007). In this project, a retired journalist visited and interviewed people aged 80 and older in Australia and New Zealand who were continuing to do remarkable things within their communities. The purpose of the research was to debunk the ageist and damaging mindset that advanced chronological age inevitably implies that an older person has become a burden on society. The revealing, and in some cases deeply personal findings, were published in a 160-page book and sent to politicians and advisers, journalists, NGOs other influential individuals, and organizations associated with ageing. The lead researcher was in her mid 70s. Her age and manner provided the necessary entrée to the private thoughts and recollections of interviewees. She found that many of the participants would not have bothered to reveal their insights to young researchers because of their perception that young westerners inadvertently display patronizing, condescending or offhand attitudes when dealing with older people.

Another study involved a virtual focus group study carried out with the assistance of nine U3A Online participants from three countries to study the successful ageing characteristics of older people who like to learn online and 'meet' like-minded virtual colleagues. The study revealed many insights, most notably the need for caution in interpreting the effects of illness and disability on perceptions of older person's abilities to continue to enjoy life. Four of the nine participants would have failed successful ageing scrutiny in terms of a narrow medical focus, yet as far as they were concerned, their quality of life was high, much of which was attributable to their daily Internet-related activities (Swindell et al. 2011).

Further details of these and other constituency research projects sponsored by U3A Online can be found at www.u3aonline.org.au.

Doubtlessly there are many examples of significant constituency research projects which have been carried out by later-life learning groups in many regions. However, the Internet has opened up a low-cost medium for research collaboration involving retired researchers. Low-cost, high-impact, collaborative constituency research projects, carried out by retired researchers from many countries, have the potential to unearth many novel findings which are beyond the reach of conventional research teams and methodologies because of constraints such as time, cost and access to participants.

The learning organizations discussed in the appendix to this chapter seem to be tailor-made for a leadership role in constituency research. These organizations are all about learning and there are few, if any, learning opportunities which can surpass discovering new knowledge or achieving novel outcomes through applied research. Although they are open to all older people, they tend to attract many with higher-than-average educational qualifications and/or those who held leadership positions in their former working lives. These are the people who could become interested in forming an international network of retired researchers who carry out research studies of benefit to the wider ageing population, nationally and internationally.

World U3A

The purpose of WorldU3A is to encourage international understanding and contacts for active retired people. It does this through its Internet activity rather than through a traditional organization structure. It has no membership and is a free service. WorldU3A evolved from the Internetwork site that was set up in 1997 to encourage Internet-based U3A networking in the UK. As U3A members from beyond the UK joined in the email discussions and started to contribute to projects, the name was changed to WorldU3A to reflect a vision of inclusivity, involving any U3A member regardless of location.

Some of the international projects carried out by email and other technology can be seen on the WorldU3A website at http://worldu3a.org. One of the most valuable of these projects is the ongoing 'technical support' email list involving a network of many U3A members with computer and Internet skills who can provide rapid answers to technology-based problems. Another is the mentoring project in which

U3A volunteers work by email with children to help them to improve their language competency. It issues a regular monthly newsletter 'Signpost' which provides links to websites of educational resources. A recent innovation is the U3A Asia Pacific Alliance. By setting up purpose-built websites WorldU3A plays an active part in the development of contacts between individual U3A members and groups in many countries, and especially in Asia and the Pacific region.

Timewitnesses

Timewitnesses, http://timewitnesses.org/, is a further example of the Internet opening up cooperative ventures for U3A members around the world. Timewitnesses is a 'living archive' which allows people from any country who have childhood or adult memories of World War II to preserve their stories for everyone. Timewitnesses is not only a powerful antiwar statement, it is an educational tool freely available to schools around the world. Many of the stories have been translated into German and French and in a number of cases school children assisted with the translations.

Conclusion

Rapid population ageing and relatively declining budgets for social services will almost inevitably result in older people having to foot considerably more of the costs associated with their own ageing. Successful ageing research suggests that the adoption of a small number of lifestyle choices by older people can maximize their chances for independence and delay or minimize the costs of expensive health and social support services in later life.

The various later-life education programmes discussed in the appendix are playing an important but largely unrecognized part in the successful ageing process. In addition, the programmes are inexpensive and uncomplicated, require little in the way of expensive infrastructure to set up and maintain, and most are situated within easy reach of the community. All contain common elements that appeal to older learners.

Although there are few obvious barriers to participation in later-life learning programmes, the total numbers of people taking part are small. For the most part, only 1–2% of the total ageing population participates. In some countries, for example China and Hong Kong, the respective governments are active in funding later-life learning programmes and encouraging older people to engage with life by taking part. In most other countries, governments are inactive in this respect. It is high time for governments everywhere to respond to the growing body of scientific evidence supporting the successful ageing elements and the positive long-term health and well-being implications for their older citizens. A 'successful ageing through later-life learning' message, coupled with funding to increase the number, range, availability and accessibility of lifelong learning programmes in local communities, particularly for older people, would be an equitable, practicable and cost-effective way of responding to the challenges of population ageing.

Appendix: Some Major Later-Life Learning Initiatives

(The principal purpose of this appendix is to provide a 2011 snapshot of major later-life learning organizations together with contact information for individuals who can provide additional details about their organizations).

University of the Third Age (U3A)

Two Universities of the Third Age Models (Adapted from Swindell and Thompson 1995)

Two distinctly different approaches to Universities of the Third Age have been successfully adopted by many countries. However, there is considerable variation within each of these approaches. The original French model (UTA) involved teaching and learning taking place in traditional university systems. In contrast, the British model, also called the self-help U3A model, which developed some years later, is run entirely by retired volunteers, often in low-cost or highly subsidized community premises, with little or no support from formal education providers. Other approaches, which incorporate some of the features of each of these 'parent' models, have evolved over the years to suit local conditions.

The French Model

An appropriate political climate for the evolution of an idea like UTA was established in France in 1968 when legislation was passed requiring universities to provide more community education. In 1973, a highly rated gerontology course, run by Toulouse University of Social Sciences exclusively for local retired people, led to the formation of the first UTA. The UTA was open to anyone over retirement age; no qualifications or examinations were required or offered, and fees were kept to a minimum. By 1975, the idea had spread to other French universities as well as to universities in Belgium, Switzerland, Poland, Italy, Spain and across the Atlantic to North America, Sherbrooke in Quebec and San Diego in California. (Despite an early introduction of UTA to the USA, the movement has not flourished there. It has been overshadowed by Lifelong Learning Institutes (LLIs) which operate in a very similar way but began a decade earlier than UTA. There is no call within the USA for a replicate later-life adult education approach).

Different UTA approaches began to develop by the late 1970s, even within France, including several which were a direct creation of local government and not connected with a university. The original focus by universities also began to broaden to include other educationally disadvantaged groups. In many places, the programmes were advertised for early retirees, housewives, the unemployed and those with disabilities. Some UTAs were renamed to reflect the changing emphasis, for example, University of Leisure Time, and Inter-Age University.

Courses vary widely in content, style of presentation and format. In general, they exhibit a mixture of open lectures, negotiated access to established university courses, and contracted courses, study groups, workshops, excursions and physical health programmes. Content is mainly in the humanities and arts. Funding also varies considerably. Some UTAs are largely university funded; some are funded by a combination of fees, donations and direct financial subsidy from the local township; and some are mainly member-funded on a sliding scale, depending on participants' assets.

The British Self-Help Model

UTA underwent a substantial change when it reached Cambridge in 1981, and the name was changed to U3A to reflect this different approach. Rather than relying on university good will, the founders of the British model adopted an approach in which there was to be no distinction between the teachers and the taught (Laslett 1989). Members would be the teachers as well as the learners and, where possible, members should engage in research activities. The 'self-help' ideal was based on the knowledge that experts of every kind retire, thus, there should be no need for older learners to have to rely on paid or unpaid Second Age teachers. Laslett provided a substantial rationale for this approach.

The self-help approach has been highly successful in Britain as well as in other countries, as described later in this appendix. Some of the strengths of the approach include: minimal membership fees; accessible classes run in community halls, libraries, private homes, schools and so forth; flexible timetables and negotiable curriculum and teaching styles; a wide course variety ranging from the highly academic to arts, crafts and physical activity; no academic constraints such as entrance requirements or examinations; and the opportunity to mix with alert like-minded people who enjoy doing new things. Each U3A is independent and is run by a democratically elected management committee of members.

IAUTA

(Contributed by Stanley Miller, past-president of IAUTA. www.aiuta.org).

The International Association of UTAs, IAUTA, which dates from 1975, was set up in order to 'federate, all over the world, Universities of the Third Age and organizations, which have different names but which subscribe to its objectives'. The principal objective is 'to constitute, with the support of Universities around the world, an international framework of a lifelong educational nature and concerned with research for, by and with the old'.

As a voluntary body, IAUTA relies heavily on the contributions of its members, individuals or Associations of UTA in more than 23 countries. Its major public function is an international congress normally held every 2 years, hosted by a member institution. IAUTA also encourages international cooperation between UTAs. For example, a study of proverbs across a number of European countries involved partners in several of those countries and culminated in two publications.

IAUTA provides a point of contact for individual UTA or UTA associations to create exchanges with fellow UTAs in other countries. Recent inquiries are leading to links between U3A in the UK and 'partner' organizations in the USA, Japan and Switzerland. The encouragement and support of U3A in different countries, both those with well-established programmes or those where the development is just beginning, is another role undertaken by IAUTA. Recently, U3A in Poland, Japan and India have all sought the help of IAUTA.

Australia and New Zealand

(Contributed by Rick Swindell, co-founder U3A Online www.u3aonline.org.au ricks1912@gmail.com).

The self-help U3A movement began in Australia in 1984 and in New Zealand in 1989. The movement spread rapidly through both countries as a 'grassroots' movement which was driven by retired community enthusiasts receiving little or no assistance from governments, NGOs or paid adult educators. By 2011 there were 240 independent U3As in Australia (69,000 members) and 65 in NZ (11,000 members). Each U3A is independent although U3A networks in the Australian States of Victoria, New South Wales, South Australia, and Queensland and in the NZ cities of Auckland, Christchurch and Wellington have considerably assisted U3A growth and development in their various regions. Since 1998, U3A Online, the world first virtual U3A, has acted as an informal network and resource centre for U3As in both countries and assisted U3A developments by providing online teaching materials and free online services which assist each U3A to better meet its educational and social objectives. In 2008, U3A Online, with three other partners, won an Australian Government $15-million bid to provide 2000 Broadband for Seniors Internet kiosks throughout Australia. This move is expected to assist with the growth and recognition of the wider U3A movement around Australia.

A U3A Australian Alliance was started several years ago, but progress has been slow. Regardless, cooperation between the various groups continues to grow, particularly through the Internet. In 2008, U3A Online funded a large scale study into the characteristics and aspirations of U3As in both countries, and the financial value of U3A volunteerism. The study was carried out by a group of eight retired U3A researchers from both countries (Swindell et al. 2009).

China

(Translated and adapted 2011 by Mr Yen Wenhui, from a speech given by Mr Yuan Xinli, President, China Association of Universities for the Aged, November 2010 AIUTA Congress).

The concept of filial piety, attributable to the great philosophy of Confucius, accounts for the respect Chinese society holds for their ageing population of 167 million people. Older people are revered for their past contributions to society as well as for their skills, wisdom and experience, which will continue to benefit the family and wider society.

The Chinese focus on lifelong learning gained strength in the 1980s, following the Cultural Revolution. Currently China has more than 40,000 U3As and more than 4.3 million older students. Government demonstrates its belief in, and commitment to the important area of elderly education, by financing most U3As.

Over the past three decades, U3A activities have evolved considerably. The first group of U3As was established mainly with an emphasis on social activities such as dancing, singing and socializing for retired officials. Now the ideas are extended much more widely into the local community with efforts made to recruit and assist older people by offering practical courses such as computer skills, English language and disease diagnosis and prevention. However, U3As are not solely places for older people to learn skills and knowledge; they also serve as important platforms for older people to contribute their expertise to wider society and to directly help others. For example, U3A members might write books, paint pictures or teach a wide range of skills. Their expertise can also extend beyond the U3A campus. For example, some members are doing voluntary work in their local communities. Others may be caring for children, passing on new knowledge or settling disputes. Still others with specific skills and knowledge are going to rural areas to disseminate their expertise in agriculture. Their contributions are widely accepted and welcomed by the communities.

In China there are three major ways to effectively utilize the experience and knowledge of the elderly people.

(a) Establishing more U3As, recruiting more students and increasing the range of subjects and interests available through the U3A curriculum. The U3A network now is spreading from the cities to the rural areas, from the central government organs to the grass-root levels.
(b) Setting up data bases for the rapid identification of older people's skills. Currently, all big cities in China have established some kind of elderly human resource database containing comprehensive details of older people's skills and experience. When an appropriate opportunity is identified, the centres recommend the employment of capable older people to positions in which they can continue to contribute to the society economically.
(c) Maintaining a favourable social environment for older people. Mass media, the Internet and the public work together to continue to build positive images of older people and their capabilities, as well as encouraging older people themselves to take steps to fully participate in the social and economic life of their communities.

Hong Kong

(Maureen Tam msltam@ied.edu.hk provides a comprehensive overview of Later-Life Learning and the Hong Kong Elder Academies in her chapter in this book entitled Active Ageing, Active Learning: Elder Learning in Hong Kong).

India

(Contributed by Dr. Sajjan Singh, Executive Chairperson Indian Society of U3As. drsajjansingh@gmail.com).

The first U3A was formed in 2007 in Rewa, India, but the concept was in vogue in ancient India. The ethos towards old age has always been a positive one. Thus the U3A concept was easily acceptable since it involves learning and teaching. To this, service was added.

The movement gathered momentum with the formation in 2008 of the Indian Society of U3As (ISU3As) which is a networking conglomerate of bodies and intellectuals working for the welfare of the elders. By 2011 there were more than 700 individual and 30 institutional members spread all over India The first landmark achievement was the successful 'World U3A Conference on Life Long Learning and Ageing With Dignity' held in 2010.

The programmes pursued by the U3As range from the 4 day reorientation programme on 'Art of Graceful Ageing' and computer training, to the various service-oriented programmes for the welfare of elders in urban and rural sectors. On line learning is not widely used but the members are well networked through 'U3A Patrika', a monthly on line newsletter, which links the U3As and highlights their various activities as well as providing news from the wider world of U3As. The urban U3As have reached out to the rural population through their teaching and service programmes but rural U3As are yet to take off. However a beginning has been made, with the infrastructure in the villages gearing up for mobile phone and internet connectivity.

Exchange visits of U3A members to countries e.g. Nepal and Mauritius have taken place. This is being encouraged Thus learners become teachers and teachers become learners with the principal objective of safeguarding the elders' interests and serving the society.

Japan

(Contributed by Akiko Tsukatani MBE, Director-General, NPO Age Concern Japan, acj.tsuka@gmail.com).

Japan is an ultra ageing society and the cost of social and medical care for older people is already a major issue affecting all members of Japanese society. It is understood that older people can and will actively continue to contribute much to society and the economy by keeping themselves both physically and mentally healthy. Through life long learning organizations they share their accumulated knowledge, skills and experiences and help each other by creating new learning communities and new social infrastructure.

During the last 30–40 years, life long education in Japan has been provided by: private companies running culture schools; U3A style gatherings run by private groups of citizens and NPOs; Senior Colleges run by local government agencies; open university type education by universities; and on line education by Nihon Hoso Kyokai (Japan Broadcasting Association).

Most of these organizations involve professional teaching and they often have rigid regulations and limited terms for learning, say 6 months to 3 years at most. U3A style education following the self-help model is a notable exception. The first Japanese U3A for older people began in Shizuoka City in 1985 under the name of 'Kiyomigata Daigakujyuku'. The members are the teachers as well as the learners, since they have considerable expertise, skills and experiences accumulated through their earlier lives. It is thought that there are now about 100 such life long learning organizations having the same concept, all with different names.

In April, 2009, NPO Age Concern Japan established the Japan U3A Federation. It registered the Japanese U3A logo, and in the same year opened U3A Osaka, which is the first self-help type directly operated by Age Concern Japan. Recently, a Tokyo lifelong learning group called 'Tokyo U3A Heart-no-kai' joined the Federation and Settsu U3A is expected to open in 2012 in Settsu City.

The Japanese style U3As, which Age Concern Japan have been sponsoring, aim to contribute to the formation of new, sustainable and activated communities through the following three approaches:

- A wide range of classes, not only university type lectures, but also cultural classes, outgoing classes, exercises, etc run by retired experts plus occasional seminars given by professional people handling specialized topics and issues
- Widening the range of learning/teaching opportunities through networking among U3As in Japan and abroad
- Community businesses and action groups will be started to act on new understanding gained through U3A classes to discuss and solve the needs and problems that local communities are faced with.

Although the brand name 'U3A' is still quite new to Japan, the self help, action oriented approach is expected to spread throughout Japan in years to come.

Nepal

(Contributed by Jeevan Raj Lohani, Coordinator, Council of U3As in Nepal http://www.u3anepal.org/ u3akathmandu@gmail.com).

U3A in Nepal started in 2006 and has since been a regular participant in international U3A events. For example it is represented on the U3A Asia Pacific Alliance, and U3A members take part in international and regional level sharing learning programmes. The 'Council of U3As in Nepal', which is a core committee representing all U3As in Nepal, was formed in 2006 and registered as a Non-Governmental Organization (NGO) in 2008. Activities within the Nepal U3A movement include (1) organization of discussion programmes, (2) supporting education related workshops, (3) forming new groups and (4) providing technical assistance to support university activities. The Council of U3As in Nepal believes key areas for Nepal and similar countries to consider are (1) financing U3As (2) adaptation of U3As in the culture of developing countries and (3) cooperation and coordination with other U3As throughout the world. Despite intense interest in modernizing and expanding U3As, the resource constraints among U3A members have limited the expansion process. In this context, the Council is seeking to promote virtual U3As among computer-literate urban populations, and sharing learning programmes among rural U3As.

North America

(Information on LLIs provided by Nancy Merz-Nordstrom, Director: Elderhostel Institute Network (EIN). Information on OLLIs provided by Kali Lightfoot, Executive Director, National Resource Center (http://www.osher.net)).

Lifelong Learning Institutes (LLIs)

(Note: The LLI movement started in 1962, about a decade before the UTA movement in France. However, because U3A is a known 'brand name' in many countries the North American approaches are discussed under the U3A heading).

Imagine a school without grades or tests, a place where the only prerequisites are an active mind and a desire to learn in a congenial atmosphere. Fill the classrooms with dedicated students of retirement age, forming a community of learners who design their own college-level curriculum according to their own needs and interests, and people whose common bonds are intellectual curiosity and the experience of their generation. They share opinions, knowledge and expertise with humour, creativity and mutual respect. When classes are over, the lively discussions don't end. The talk spills out to the hallways, the cafeteria or the student lounge. Younger students passing through are impressed by the vitality of this enthusiastic bunch. Learning through the LLI movement in North America is fun and appealing to rapidly growing numbers of older learners.

The first LLIs trace their roots back to 1962 when the Institute for Retired Professionals was started in New York City under the sponsorship of the New School for Social Research. During the next 26 years, until the formation of the Elderhostel

Institute Network in 1988, the idea spread relatively slowly, primarily by word of mouth with little media attention. By 1988 there were about 50 separate LLI groups. In 2011, there were almost 400 programmes, the majority affiliated with higher education institutions but also programmes connected with active retirement communities, senior centres, community organizations and even some 'stand-alone' programmes with no affiliation whatsoever. Keeping older adults active, involved and contributing to society in mind, body and spirit are the major goals.

LLIs are known by many names, with each being a unique organization reflecting the needs and goals of its sponsoring campus and participants from the local community. Several years ago many of the current LLIs changed their name from Institutes for Learning in Retirement because market surveys showed that young North American retirees do not want to join organizations labelled as being for retirees.

Elderhostel

In 1975 the Elderhostel organization was formed to provide short, university-based adult education courses for older adults. The concept involved inviting older adults from anywhere in the USA to live as students on a university campus for about a week during student vacations, to take intensive mini-courses, usually taught by paid members of the faculty. Elderhostel is a not-for-profit organization. However costs must be covered and course participants are required to pay for travel, accommodation, teaching fees and other expenses associated with their week of study at a distant campus. The fees would deter many would-be older learners with limited resources. Despite this, the programmes are very popular with older adults and Elderhostel is now the world's largest, educational travel organization.

In 1988, 24 LLIs collaborated with Elderhostel to form the Elderhostel Institute Network (EIN), with a mission to strengthen and support the effectiveness of both programmes and spread the LLI concept to new communities. The EIN has been effective at promoting the rapid growth of LLIs in both the USA and Canada.

Osher Lifelong Learning Institutes (OLLIs)

The Bernard Osher Foundation was founded in 1977 by a prominent California businessman seeking to improve quality of life through support for higher education and the arts. In 2001, the Foundation began to support university-based programmes targeted toward more mature students through grants to both startup and existing lifelong learning institutes. OLLIs operate in a way similar to the LLIs outlined above, and many OLLIs started as LLIs before receiving Osher funding. In 2011, there were 118 OLLIs operating in all 50 USA States. Like the LLIs there is considerable variation among the OLLIs (the Osher Foundation is non-prescriptive and interested in supporting a wide array of programme models) but the common threads remain: Non-credit educational programmes specifically developed for adults who are aged 50 and older; university connection and university support; robust volunteer leadership and sound organizational structure; and a diverse repertoire of intellectually stimulating courses. In 2004, the Osher Foundation endowed the National Resource Center (NRC) for OLLIs at the University of Southern Maine. The NRC organizes national conferences for the network of OLLIs, and provides a communication hub and repository of promising practices by and for staff and volunteer leaders of the OLLIs, LLIs and other learning organizations. The NRC website: http://www.osher.net will give the reader a taste of the variety of classes, special events and projects being offered at the OLLIs, as well as resources available to anyone interested in creating an educational programme aimed at older adults.

Republic of South Africa

(Contributed by Kathrine Fenton-May, Durban U3A, kathrine@iafrica.com).

The first U3A (self-help model) started in 2000 in Cape Town. By 2011, 25 independent groups with a combined total of about 8,000 members were providing a diverse range of courses in five of the nine provinces. There are 11 official languages in the republic of South Africa. However, the U3A groups are mainly English speaking and have not yet started in regions where English is not widely spoken. A number of U3As have some members from the other indigenous cultures. In the Western Cape area, five of the groups get together at a Forum which increases communications and exchange of ideas.

SACE-U3A Singapore

(Contributed by Thomas Kuan, past-president of the Singapore Association for Continuing Education (www.sace.org.sg); chair, University of the Third Age Asia Pacific Alliance. kuanthomas@gmail.com).

The Singapore Association for Continuing Education (SACE) plays an overarching role in the development of continuing education in Singapore. In 2006, in line with one of its objectives 'to encourage interest in and support for the development of continuing education' the first Singapore U3A was formed. SACE-U3A activities are organized on the British model where members volunteer their time and share their expertise with other members and their friends. SACE's most recent major regional leadership activities include membership of the University of the Third Age Asia Pacific Alliance, and organization of the 2011 International U3A Conference in Singapore.

United Kingdom

(Contributed by Ian Searle, Chairman of the Third Age Trust. www.u3a.org.uk).

The British model of U3A was started in 1982 when the first local groups were set up. In the absence of support from Universities or Adult Education authorities, members themselves ran interest groups and meetings, often in each others' homes. The Third Age Trust and National Office were set up to support new groups and to circulate a news sheet. At the beginning of 2011, there were 782 local U3As with very nearly 250,000 members. Each U3A is operationally independent but has corporate membership of the Third Age Trust. With the Trust's support Subject Networks were set up to link and encourage new groups in such subjects as Languages, Music and Science. The 34 Coordinators offer support and some also organize newsletters, Study Days and sometimes residential courses. The quarterly magazine, 'U3A News' is now posted directly to most members' homes and it is accompanied by the educational journal 'Sources', written by members.

In the past 2 years, there has been increased emphasis on the development of regional committees to encourage and assist development. The Trust is administered by 12 Regional Trustees, one elected from each of the English Regions and one each from Northern Ireland, Scotland and Wales. There are a further four elected Officers. Joint U3A activities and get-togethers for special occasions are increasing. Opportunities for members to meet and share ideas flourish at the biannual Conference and the AGM, arranged by the Trust each September, as well as at the popular residential Summer Schools.

For some years now the Third Age Trust has joined U3A Online to supply online courses from both organizations to both the UK and elsewhere. A UK Virtual U3A with its own interest groups has recently started and is now a member of the Trust.

Memoranda of Understanding have been agreed with the Open University and with the Workers Educational Association. Guest speakers from both organizations contribute to various meetings and it is hoped to make increasing use of the Open Learn material from the OU. Furthermore annual events are organized with the Royal Institution and with DANA at which eminent researchers into Science and Neuroscience speak to U3A members. An annual Science Conference is arranged in Abergavenny, Wales.

There has been notable progress in recent years in the UK in obtaining public recognition for the work of U3As. In 2008, the Third Age Trust was invited to participate in a government-sponsored series of discussions on the subject of non-formal adult education. That led to the publication of 'Time to Learn', an exposition of the U3A methodology. In partnership with the National Institute for Adult and Continuing Education, the same information was used to produce a new website www.selforganisedlearning.org.uk. Close liaison with many other organizations has followed and the Trust's views are now often solicited on matters to do with older people's learning. A Research Committee is currently seeking closer links with a wide range of UK universities to work in partnership. The employment of a professional educational journalist has greatly enhanced the public awareness of the U3A movement and its achievements, and press releases are issued frequently. The national website, www.u3a.org.uk, provides much more information and is heavily used by both U3A members and interested visitors. The Trust has also sponsored the production of a great deal of information and publicity material, and a professionally made DVD is shortly to be released. A short history of the U3A movement in the UK was also commissioned in 2010.

On the international scene, the Trust is represented on IAUTA. From 2007 to 2011, the IAUTA President was a former Vice Chairman of the Third Age Trust. Another Vice Chairman was invited as a guest speaker to a conference of Hong Kong U3As in 2007, and the Trust sent a representative to the conference in Chikrakoot in 2010, and to Singapore in 2011.

U3A in Brief in Some Other Countries

(Contributed by Stanley Miller, past-president of the International Association of Universities of the Third Age. www.aiuta.org).

Belgium – French speaking Belgium was one of the earliest in the development of UTAs beyond France. It has two very active UTAs in Louvain-la-Neuve (not Louvain/Leuven) and Namur. The former, with its various branches in Brussels and in other parts of that region has around 5–6,000 members. The Namur UTA has been involved in a great deal of cooperative work with U3As in other countries, as well as in some interesting community and intergenerational work.

Canada – Different later-life learning programmes operate in francophone and anglophone Canada . In the former, Sherbrooke, Quebec and Montreal are important centres of U3A activity. In the latter, U3As as such do not exist; instead U3A style learning and teaching activities are run under different names (e.g. LLIs, OLLIs). There is a federation/network (CATALIST) but, so far, they have shown little international activity.

Czech Republic – There is a federation comprising some 35 U3As.

France – In addition to the following list of U3As, there is a federation UFUTA (The French Union of U3As with about 42 members). Toulouse, Vannes, Versailles, Lyon, Creteil, Limoges, Paris 6, Rheims, Orleans, Lille, Melun, Evry, Lannion plus two in overseas 'departments' –Martinique and Noumea. There is also the worldwide francophone welfare association, FIAPA, which brings together national associations, of which IAUTA is part.

Finland – Joensuu, Jyväskylä, Helsinki.

Germany – The U3A title is not used in Germany although there are a number of organizations operating in a similar vein within an overall organization concerned for the welfare of older people (BAGSO). (This situation also applies in other European contexts e.g. Spain with FATEC which is a Catalan Federation). The University of Ulm Centre for Academic Research (ZAWIW) is an internationally renowned centre in the field of e-learning for seniors.

Greece – An organization in Athens called 50 plus embraces the U3A concept.

Italy – At least two large federations of U3As: UNITRE is based in Turin and FEDERUNI, which is largely based on universities with an interest in lifelong learning. More than 100 U3As belong to UNITRE.

Luxemburg – At least one at Ettelbruch.

Malta – based in Valetta and the university is much involved in gerontological studies.

Netherlands – Gronigen and Nijmegen, both now represented on the IAUTA Governing Board.

Norway – PUNR (Pensjonistuniversitetet Dedre Romerike) which is an independent U3A organization established in 1993 for the geographical area of Nedre Romerike, north of Oslo. In 2006, there were about 500 members.

Poland – Two U3As in Warsaw, one of which, MUTW, does considerable supportive work on behalf of Polish-speaking U3As in Moldavia, Belarus and the Ukraine. There is also a long-standing U3A at the University of Lublin.

Portugal – The total number of U3As in 2011 may be close to 100. There is a U3A federation called RUTIS.

Slovakia – The Comenius University of Bratislava has an active centre for U3A work. This U3A is also part of a partnership based on the river Danube and the countries through which it flows.

Spain – U3As operate in Seville, Alicante, Santiago de Compestella, Madrid, Seville, Grenada, Santander, La Coruna, Barcelona (Catalan) as well as expatriate U3As for British and French living in retirement in Spain. There are also federations APFA/AFOPA and UNATE, which, in the latter case, is again a general welfare organization but with a learning strand.

Sweden – U3As in Gotenberg and Uppsala.

Switzerland – U3As in Lucerne, Basle, Berne, Giubiasco, Lausanne, Neuchatel, Zurich and Geneva, the latter a particularly internationally oriented U3A.

Latin America – U3As are found in Argentina, Chile, Brazil, Colombia and Costa Rica. These are largely individual U3As based on universities.

References

Andel, R., Crowe, M., Pedersen, N. L., Fratiglioni, L., Johansson, B., & Gatz, M. (2008). Physical exercise at midlife and risk of dementia three decades later: A population-based study of Swedish twins. *Journals of Gerontology Series A-Biological Sciences & Medical Sciences, 63*(1), 62–66.

Barron, S., Tan, E., Yu, Q., Song, M., McGill, S., & Fried, L. (2009, July). Potential for intensive volunteering to promote the health of older adults in fair health. *Journal of Urban Health, 86*(4), 641–653. Published online 2009 June 2. doi: 10.1007/s11524-009-9353-8. PMCID: PMC2704275.

Beddington, J., Cooper, C., Field, J., Goswami, U., Huppert, F., Jenkins, R., Jones, H., Kirkwood, T., Sahakian, B., & Thomas, S. (2008). The mental wealth of nations. *Nature, 455*(7216), 1057–1060.

Bowling, A. (1994). Social networks and social support among older people and implications for emotional well-being and psychiatric morbidity. *International Review of Psychiatry, 6*, 41–58.
Braxton, D., Swindell, R., & MacKinlay, E. (2007). *A voice worth listening to*. Charnwood: Ginninderra Press.
Dorling, D., Vickers, D., Thomas, B., Pritchard, J., & Ballas, D. (2008). *Changing UK: The way we live now*. Retrieved February 21, 2011, from http://sasi.group.shef.ac.uk/research/changingUK.html
Erickson, K., Raji, C., Lopez, O., Becker, J., Rosano, C., Newman, A., & Kuller, L. (2010, October 19). Physical activity predicts gray matter volume in late adulthood: The cardiovascular health study. *Neurology*, *75*(16), 1415–1422.
Erikson, K., Voss, M., Prakash, R., Basak, C., Szabo, A., Chaddock, L., & Kramer, A. F. (2011). Exercise training increases size of hippocampus and improves memory. *Proceedings of the National Academy of Sciences of the United States of America, 108*(7), 3017–3022. doi:10.1073/pnas.1015950108.
Ertel, K., Glymour, M., & Berkman, L. (2008). Effects of social integration on preserving memory function in a nationally representative U.S. elderly population. *American Journal of Public Health, 98*(7), 1215–20.
Friedrich, D. (2003). Personal and societal intervention strategies for successful ageing. *Ageing International, 28*(1), 3–36.
Glass, T. (2003). Successful aging. In R. Talli, H. Fillit, & J. C. Brocklehurst (Eds.), *Brocklehurst's textbook of geriatric medicine and gerontology* (6th ed.). London: Churchill Livingstone.
Harper, S. (2008). *Generations and life course: The impact of demographic challenges on education 2010–2050*. Retrieved February 22, 2011, from, http://www.ageing.ox.ac.uk/system/files/publication_challenges_on_education_2010–2050.pdf
House, J., Landis, K., & Umberson, D. (1988). Social relationships and health. *Science, 241*, 540–545.
LARA Learning a response to Ageing. (n.d.). Retrieved February 21, 2011, from, http://www.laraproject.net/images/stories/lara/pdf/lara%20research%20report-1.pdf
Laslett, P. (1989). *A fresh map of life*. London: Weidenfeld and Nicolson.
Lautenschlager, N., Cox, K., Flicker, L., Foster, J., van Bockxmeer, F., Xiao, J., Greenop, K., & Almeida, O. (2008). Effect of physical activity on cognitive function in older adults at risk for Alzheimer disease: A randomized trial. *Journal of the American Medical Association, 300*(9), 1027–1037.
Madden, M. (2010). *Older adults and social media. Pew internet and American life project*. Retrieved February 21, 2011, from, http://www.pewinternet.org/Reports/2010/Older-Adults-and-Social-Media.aspx
McNair, S. (2009). *Demography and lifelong learning IFLL thematic paper 1*. Retrieved February 22, 2011, from http://shop.niace.org.uk/ifll-demography-freedownload.html
Productivity Commission. (2010). *Caring for older Australians* (Draft Inquiry Report, Canberra). Retrieved February 22, 2011, from http://www.pc.gov.au/projects/inquiry/aged-care/draft
Rainee, L., Purcell, K., & Smith, A. (2011). *The social side of the internet. Pew internet and American life project*. Retrieved February 21, 2011, from http://www.pewinternet.org/Press-Releases/2011/Social-Side-of-the-Internet.aspx
Rowe, J., & Kahn, R. (1999). *Successful aging*. New York: Random House.
Schuller, T., & Watson, D. (n.d.). *Learning through life: Easy read summary*. Retrieved February 23, 2011, from http://shop.niace.org.uk/media/catalog/product/f/i/file_3_24.pdf
Small, G., Moody, T., Siddarth, P., & Bookheimer, S. (2009). Your brain on google: Patterns of cerebral activation during internet searching. *The American Journal of Geriatric Psychiatry, 17*(2), 116–126.
Smith, J., Nielson, K., Woodard, J., Seidenberg, M., Durgerian, S., Antuono, P., & Rao, S. (2011). Interactive effects of physical activity and APOE-ε4 on BOLD semantic memory activation in healthy elders. *NeuroImage, Jan 1;54*(1), 635–44.
Soar, J., Swindell, R., & Tsang, P. (Eds.). (2011). *Intelligent technologies for bridging the grey digital divide*. Hershey: Information Science Reference.

Swindell, R., & Mayhew, C. (1996). Educating the isolated ageing: Improving the quality of life of the housebound elderly through educational teleconferencing. *International Journal of Lifelong Education, 15*(2), 85–93.

Swindell, R., & Thompson, J. (1995). An international perspective of the University of the Third Age. *Educational Gerontology, 21*(5), 429–447.

Swindell, R., James, C., & Mann, M. (1992). *A study of teleconferencing as a medium for improving the quality of life of the frail elderly* (ERIC Document Reproduction Service No. ED 346 310).

Swindell, R., Singer, L., & Singer, G. (1994). Teleconferencing as a medium for providing expert support to the isolated ageing. *Australian Journal on Ageing, 13*(2), 93–94.

Swindell, R., Vassella, K., Morgan, L., & Sayer T. (2009). *U3As in Australia and New Zealand 2008: The successful ageing organisations* (Eric Document Reproduction Service No. ED507026).

Swindell, R., Grimbeek, P., & Heffernan, J. (2011). U3A online and successful aging: A smart way to help bridge the grey digital divide. In J. Soar, R. Swindell, & P. Tsang (Eds.), *Intelligent technologies for bridging the grey digital divide* (pp. 122–140). Hershey: Information Science Reference.

The Research Council of Norway. (2010, November 27). Elderly to outnumber children by 2050 in most parts of world. *ScienceDaily*. Retrieved February 23, 2011, from http://www.sciencedaily.com/releases/2010/11/101126094441.htm

Vaillant, G. (2002). *Aging well.* New York: Little, Brown.

Wrosch, C., & Schulz, R. (2008). Health-engagement control strategies and 2-year changes in older adults' physical health. *Psychological Science, 19*(6), 537–541.

Zedlewski, S., & Butrica, B. (2007). *Are we taking full advantage of older adults potential? Perspectives on productive aging, The Urban Institute* (Number 9, December). Retrieved February 23, 2011, from http://www.urban.org/UploadedPDF/411581_adult_potential.pdf

Swindell, R., & Mayhew, C. (1996). Educating the isolated ageing: Improving the quality of life of the housebound elderly through educational teleconferencing. *International Journal of Lifelong Education, 15*(2), 85–93.

Swindell, R., & Thompson, J. (1995). An international perspective on the University of the Third Age. *Educational Gerontology, 21*(5), 429–447.

Swindell, R., [illegible] C., & [illegible] M. ([illegible]). *A study of teleconference* [illegible] [illegible]

Part II
Research Methods on Ageing Issues

Chapter 5
Using Narrative Inquiry and Analysis of Life Stories to Advance Elder Learning

Nancy Lloyd Pfahl

Introduction

Learning is a lifelong process of connection, reexamination, and change (Cross 1999). When we reflect cognitively to create narratives that story life experience, "… human organisms make meaning" (Kegan 1994, p. 29) of experience by attending to it and learning from it. When we think about *how* and *why* events have happened, narrative becomes the form of examination with potential to answer such questions, to expand our understanding, and to influence and change our patterns of thought and action.

On the other hand, if life stagnates, we can become immobilized, unable to see alternatives and connections among our experiences; we then risk regressive thought and behavior patterns. It seems reasonable to assume that relational narrative thinking plays a significant role in recharging our motivations and brains and in expanding perception throughout life. It is the natural means for elder learners to address challenges of changing as they age and of integrating life experience to pass on wisdom to younger generations. If narrative weaves the threads of life into the fabric of experience, how can educators use narrative processes to expand the learning potential of increasingly elder audiences? How can stories of our elders enrich the quality of family relationships, institutions, and communities?

During much of the twentieth century, we emphasized paradigmatic, linear thought over relational thinking (Bruner 1985a, b). This choice devalued the influence of context and encouraged examining phenomena in isolation, a logical consequence of the scientific method. Assume for the moment that (1) we learn in order to develop and change as we age; (2) construct our realities in response to our learning

N.L. Pfahl (✉)
Adult Learning and Resource Development Consultant, 1511 Portner Road,
Alexandria, VA 22314, USA
e-mail: nlpfahl@earhlink.net

G.M. Boulton-Lewis and M. Tam (eds.), *Active Ageing, Active Learning: Issues and Challenges*, Education in the Asia-Pacific Region: Issues, Concerns and Prospects 15,
DOI 10.1007/978-94-007-2111-1_5,

and stage of development; and (3) use narrative processes, often without awareness or intent. If these assumptions are valid, then there is learning potential in narrating experience, collecting its stories, and analyzing them to interpret and create reality and the self and to understand *how* and *why* to revise unproductive patterns of behavior.

The preceding assumptions resonate in *Love in the Time of Cholera* (Márquez 1988). This novel traces the life experiences of two ageing men living in the same village. His story of their lives depicts dramatic differences in their capacities to learn, their developmental stages, and their interpretations of the changing world order. Florentino defies convention and retains his vitality as a man willing to begin anew regardless of ageing, love, and circumstance, while Juvenal Urbino relinquishes all opportunities for love and growth. Florentino fulfills his uncle's narrative conviction "that human beings are not born once…but that life obliges them over and over again to give birth to themselves" (p. 165). In turn, the reader is offered a door through which to achieve hope, a creation of meaning.

Didion (1979) remarks similarly to Márquez's narrative: "We tell ourselves stories in order to live…we interpret what we see, select the most workable of the multiple choices. We live entirely…by the imposition of a narrative line upon disparate images, by the 'ideas' with which we have learned to freeze the phantasmagoria, which is our actual experience" (p. 11).

Precisely through narratives, Márquez and Didion raise the questions: How can we understand, structure, and augment our own thinking in order to achieve longer, higher-quality lives? Secondly, how can this learning evolution be addressed and capitalized upon by applying narrative inquiry and analysis to life experience during a rapidly changing new century?

Defining Narrative, Narrative Inquiry, and Narrative Analysis

Throughout all cultures, the pervasiveness of narrative processes, particularly storytelling, speaks to learning from experience (Cell 1984). Narrative, a "root metaphor" (Pepper 1942 as cited in Sarbin 1986, p. 1) for life experience, can bridge isolated events, learning and longevity challenges, and societal shifts and trends. It is a venue for conveying how differences, separations, and unions of opposing elements can form new understanding that crosses boundaries. Embedded in stories of experience are values and emotions, wedded to context and meaning, that inform narrative interpretation and societal complexity. Attending to inductive narrative processes offers a relational approach that complements deductive, analytical thinking. Using *both* forms of thought as complements creates a more holistic learning strategy for understanding postmodern life.

The term "narrative" applies to both processes and products. Clandinin and Connelly (1991) distinguish between *narrative* and *story*. They use *narrative* in reference to the process of inquiry and *story* in reference to the phenomenon, understanding "narrative as both phenomena under study and method of study" (Clandinin and Connelly 2000, p. 3). Thus, we say that "people by nature lead storied lives and tell stories of those lives, whereas narrative researchers describe such lives, collect and tell stories of them, and write narratives of experience" (Clandinin and Connelly 1991, p. 2). There is, however, lack of agreement about the terminology. In ordinary usage, we define *narrative* as synonymous with *story*. In the latter view, a narrative can be a story that reconstructs lived experience. In either case, narrative requires reflecting on lived experience and integrating various elements of narrative schema, including time, context (setting), and action (plot) that engages actors (characters) distinguished by voice, knowledge, skills, attitudes, values, emotions, beliefs, somatic sensing, and imagination. Narration that incorporates this synthesis focuses on action, provides a means for reflection, and contributes to constructing the self.

Narrative inquiry, a discipline within the broader field of qualitative research, is a way of understanding and researching how people make meaning of their storied lives. It offers a natural, human approach to research, for humans exhibit what Bruner (1990) has called protolinguistic readiness to organize experience relationally. Narrative inquiry offers a compatible way to study narrative processes (Clandinin and Connelly 2000) by collecting a repertory of indigenous stories to (1) communicate both tacit and explicit ideas to others and (2) discover new meaning by "assimilating experiences into narrative schema" (Gudmundsdottir 1995, p. 34). By accessing a repertory of related stories from a group of elder learners, narrative research has the power to bring the meanings of the participants' individual stories into a broader context, transforming both the participants as co-researchers and their interpretations of the stories (Schaafsma 1993).

A strong, multidimensional basis for narrative thinking integrates personal history and societal change, part of the trend toward integration rather than separation. Narrative inquiry draws upon memory, making connections between the conscious and the subconscious and between past and present. By triggering memory, narrative inquiry and analysis seem particularly relevant to studying elder learners engaged in life review. This methodology prompts elder learners and research-oriented educators as interpreters, artists, and composers (Price 1999), for variables cannot be identified easily and examining life experience requires exploration in a natural setting (Cresswell 1994). Given a research purpose, for example, to examine the contribution of narrative to the learning and change of elder learners in context, narrative inquiry is a powerful way to interpret the *how* and the *why* of relationships among actors and events for the purpose of the participants' understanding better *how* and *why* their lives have unfolded as they have and whether and how to change outdated thought and behavior patterns.

Equally important, narrative inquiry lends itself to studying tacit, rather than explicit, knowledge (Polanyi 1966). According to Polanyi (1966), "we can know more than we can tell" (p. 4). Participants in a narrative inquiry likely will be surprised by some of the content in the stories they tell because narrative processes are largely intuitive. People are often not fully aware of the extent to which they use them. Consequently, sometimes cognitive and behavioral narrative processes have remained unidentified by name.

Dependent upon the research purpose, narrative analysis can draw upon multiple traditions of inquiry to interpret and analyze a repertoire of stories of lived experience – case study, ethnography, phenomenology, phenomenography, and various forms of literary analysis. Narrative analysis includes at least two critical dimensions: emergent story themes and recurrent patterns of action. Narrative does not lead to scientific truth, but rather establishes *lifelikeness* or *verisimilitude* (Mishler 1986) where differing, even "contradictory systems" (Kegan 2000, p. 68) and interpretations co-exist. If "truth" is sought, narrative is not the process for finding it, for it is an interpretative process.

Learning in a Networked Context

Global networking is accelerating the process of connecting and unifying differences across spatial and chronological boundaries to produce a sense of presence long distance. Integration has brought together learning and development, until recently considered by many to be two separate disciplines (Merriam 2001). The trends toward networking and integrating learning and development suggest that networks of connection, both electronic and interdisciplinary, inform learning, shape development, influence our actions, and expand our capacity to rewrite the self (Freeman 1993), our institutions, and society.

Learning involves "taking apart and putting together the structures that give our lives meaning" (Daloz 1986, p. 236). This very construction and deconstruction is the essence of the Internet and digital era. Identifying patterns of lived experience holds the ability to transform experience (Daloz 1986; Kegan 1994, 2000). How can "hits" and "connections" of Facebook-esque digital social networking be used to increase learning and other capacity potentials of an ageing population, potentials reaching far beyond the commercial marketing realm? How do they impact their stories of experience?

As people are living increasingly longer lives, this "longevity revolution" requires "a new distribution of the stages of life" (Boia 2004, p. 177). Meaningfulness changes at different times of life, a result of learning or not learning from experience to foster or suppress development. Identity is the consequence of both. Piaget (1955) contended that a child develops while learning through social interaction, a premise that now is held true for adults (Kegan 1994; Merriam and Clark 2006; Clark and Rossiter 2008; Taylor and Lamaroux 2008). This reciprocity depends upon (1) learning processes that constitute development and (2) development that organizes and structures learning processes (Keller and Werchan 2006).

Bateson (2010) describes Adulthood II, ages 50–75, as an art form requiring improvisation and willingness to learn. Exploring connections among life experiences leads older adults to a capacity for *wisdom*, a higher level of integration, characterized by integrity rather than isolation and despair of death. Body, mind, and emotion function as an integrated learning system that relies upon interaction among (1) *context*, (2) *community*, (3) *cognitive reflection* [that encompasses *rational reflection* and *narrative refraction*, Pfahl 2003], (4) *somatic reflection*, and (5) *time* (Merriam and Clark 2006).

Context

Contextual learning places information and knowledge within an environment similar to narrative setting. A global exploration of fables, for example, reveals how ancient constructions, orchestrated to shape culture, have fostered the evolution of daily existence. Regardless of being absorbed actively or without awareness or intent, fables and other kinds of story help to derive individual, community, and global meaning from the past, present, and future. How can elder learners be guided to reconstruct their life stories and identities to discover renewed meaning in life toward the enhancement of community and global change? An active longevity potential allows society to learn from experience, to grasp a multiplicity of opportunities, and to deepen intergenerational connectedness.

Community

Actively ageing in a continuously changing, diversified world prompts adults to see themselves, others, knowledge, feelings, communication styles, and morals as elements of a complex system where reconciliation of difference *is* possible. By intentionally storying and opening one's personal value system, a new system can emerge that incorporates a multiplicity of individual, community, and societal values. Differences co-exist more amicably in a more inclusive, integrated state of development (Kegan 1994). Under these circumstances, learning, an active, socially constructed process, takes place in community (Merriam and Clark 2006), with different learning and development possibilities arising during dialogue and narration.

In a learning group and at the team level, "learning involves the mutual construction of new knowledge, including the capacity for concerted collaborative action" (Marsick and Watkins 2001, p. 32). A functional community, "where common ground can be found where all contending 'cultures' can stand together in wholeness and distinctness" (Kegan 1994, p. 345), enables people to engage in informal give-and-take. Mutual construction of knowledge requires listening for difference, supporting collaboration rather than competition, providing support toward action and achievement, and deconstructing outdated narratives and constructing revised scenarios. Cultural beliefs, attitudes, values, and social mores inform experiential stories and create synergy where each person's unique lens of experience, informed by stage of development, plays a role in interpretation.

Cognitive Reflection

Dialogical processes are narrative in nature. Differing perspectives coming together in dialogue advance connected knowing and cognitive development (Belenky and

Stanton 2000). Given that we learn from difference, sharing and interpreting experience with others is helpful in transitioning individual experience from *subject* to *object* within a group context (Kegan 2000). Examining experience cognitively as *object* to interpret the interaction between learning and development takes two different forms: *rational reflection* – critically reflective paradigmatic thinking that is logical (Merriam and Clark 2006) – and what the learning model names and describes as *narrative refraction* – viewing experience through a wide-angle lens and interpreting it relationally, thinking and acting toward broadened contextual understanding and knowing (Pfahl 2003). Rational reflection and narrative refraction enable us to consider life experience from two different points of view: evaluative and interpretative. When each mode of thought informs the other, we learn more holistically, expanding our understanding of the socio-cultural contexts that influence our knowing and development.

Somatic Reflection

Emotion impacts our reasoning and prompts somatic input that provides a different form of reflection communicated through anatomical responses. Somatic reflection prompts sudden "gut reactions," often appearing without anticipation. Gut reactions trigger responses that are indispensable to rationalism: "Feelings point us in the proper direction, take us to an appropriate place in a decision-making space, where we may put the instruments of logic to good use" (Demasio 1994, as cited in Dowling 1998, p. 175).

Time

Learning through reflection requires time; development advances or regresses through time; and time structures narrative, just as narrative structures experience. Time orders life experience and narrative action (Polkinghorne 1988) by embodying the "emergence of newness, a sense of becoming" (Jarvis 2006), for time does not stand still. In maximizing our learning and longevity potentials, we are in a continuous process of becoming something other, recreating our identities as we accumulate temporal experience in storied form. As life unfolds in community, and as we learn from the experience of others, our identities develop, and we become better positioned to revise our thoughts and actions.

Narrative Learning Model

Human interaction evolves naturally as narrative plot. Using narrative processes is a formative part of our being, but frequently we are unaware of using them as learning strategies; then the processes remain unnamed. Narrative processes are "hermeneutic

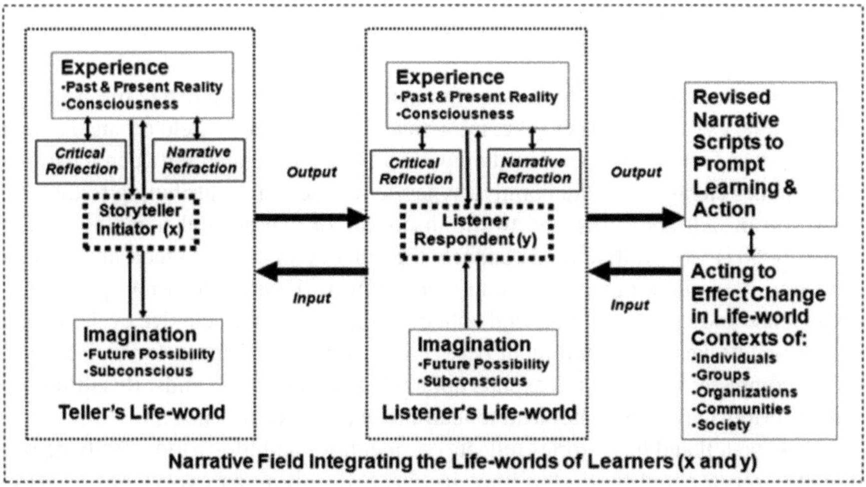

Fig. 5.1 Learning and changing: Interaction between a storyteller and a listener in a narrative field that integrates their life-worlds (Revision based upon Pfahl 2003 © Nancy Lloyd Pfahl 2009)

processes of relational thinking that foster the emergence of story and draw upon context and difference as interpretative means for learning from lived experience" (Pfahl 2003, p. 508). Storytelling, scenario building, questioning, and integration, for example, take both cognitive and behavioral forms. The cognitive, previously identified as characteristic of team learning but not as narrative processes, includes framing, reframing, and integrating perspectives, (Kasl et al. 1997), as well as creating memory (Pfahl 2003). Linked behaviors dependent upon relational and inductive thinking include experimenting and crossing boundaries (Kasl et al. 1997), as well as narrative inquiry, collaboration, and process improvement (Pfahl 2003). Narrative processes are dynamic elements of incidental learning that "may be taken for granted, tacit, or unconscious" (Marsick and Watkins 2001, p. 26). Informal learning, often the by-product of other activity, "rests primarily in the hands of the learner" (p. 25).

Narrative is a bridge connecting multiple interpretations of experience to learning; as assumptions change, learning can occur and consciousness expand. Narrative thinking can motivate adults, unlock their learning potential, and prompt them to rewrite scripts for the future (Pfahl and Wiessner 2007; Wiessner and Pfahl 2007). In this process, the brain uses analogy to connect new input to existing patterns (Taylor and Lamaroux 2008). Actions may change these patterns or not, for we are shaped by what we do. Constructing life stories requires intentionality; involves collaborative action and mediation of attitudes, beliefs, emotions, and values in context; and reflects level of learning and stage of development.

Figure 5.1 illustrates narrative interaction that occurs in daily conversation: story construction combining conscious experiential reality and subconscious imagination. By contrast to community-based and informal lifelong learning in non-Western cultures, "most Westerners neither recognize nor value learning that is embedded in everyday life" (Merriam and Kim 2008, p. 75).

Narrative Field

Figure 5.1 illustrates social processes of narrative learning in contextual life-worlds of a storyteller (x) and a listener (y) communicating in a narrative field of engagement. A *narrative field* is "the perceived empathic energy generated between a narrator and listener engaged in collaborative synergic interactions contributing to the construction of *self* and *other* and to the discovery of experiential meaning" (Pfahl 2003, p. 507). A narrative field connects the teller and listener to tacit and somatic knowing. Recounting an experiential story informs them by drawing upon shared experience and upon individual and collective imagination. Recursive cycles evolve as give-and-take, output and input between the teller and listener, for their story is never complete; its meaning depends upon where it begins and ends. Resulting narrative scripts may or may not lead to learning and revised action.

How we tell and hear stories reflects our identities and life-worlds. Both are permeable, represented by dotted lines in Fig. 5.1. Telling an experience accesses subconscious possibilities and draws upon individual life-world experience, consciousness, and imagination. A teller integrates input from different aspects of knowing, combining relational input from narrative refraction, factual information derived from critical thinking, tacit knowledge of the subconscious, and somatic input. The teller integrates these contributing elements in story as narrative output to the listener, thereby becoming part of the listener's experience. The listener then becomes the teller, sharing a reinterpretation as new input to the original teller. Thus, the listener's response can become a trigger for the teller to remember more details and possibly to change perspective. Dependent upon the teller's reactions to alternative interpretations, outcomes can range from learning and reconstruction of new meaning to inaction and unwillingness to acknowledge difference or to change.

Storying and Restorying Experience

Part of the significance of narrating experience lies in connecting the conscious and subconscious by using narrative processes to surface tacit knowledge (Polyani 1966). Figure 5.2 interprets patterns of interaction between teller and listener: When two life-worlds connect to inform experience, the connection prompts reinterpretation of experience and deconstruction and reconstruction of reality.

In narrative inquiry, a research participant (x_1) tells a story of experience related to the interview topic. The researcher (y_2) records the interview, listens, reflects, and interprets the participant's story through his or her lens of personal experience. The researcher then reconstructs the story from the interview text, retelling or writing the reinterpretation (y_3) for the participant (x_4) to reconsider. Reading or listening to the researcher's reinterpretation of the original story, reflecting and reinterpreting it again brings forth the participant's tacit knowledge and additional

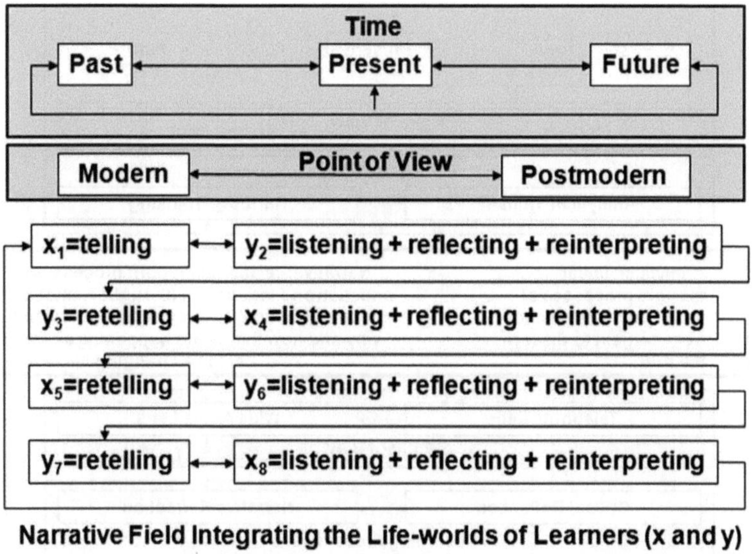

Fig. 5.2 Storying and restorying experience: Interaction between a storyteller (x) and a listener (y) interpreting the meaning of experience in a narrative field by telling, listening, reflecting, reinterpreting, and retelling experience (Revision based upon Pfahl 2003 © Nancy Lloyd Pfahl 2009)

detail stored in subconscious memory but not remembered at the time of the first telling. Then the participant's reinterpretation of the original story, interpreted during a second interview through the lens of the researcher's experience, informs the interview and provides an expanded version of the story (x_5), reinterpreted for a second time by the researcher (y_6). Each successive restorying and reinterpretation of the original story prompts additional memories in preparation for their next interchange and its subsequent learning cycle. When we narrate experience within a recursive system as described above, retelling is a natural consequence of dialogue that incorporates collaborative reflection between co-learners engaged in narrative inquiry, as in a series of conversations, dialogues, or interviews. Conducting multiple interviews over time with the same participant reveals the participant's unexpected recounting of subconscious tacit knowledge during the telling (Pfahl 2003).

Differentiating Critical Reflection and Narrative Refraction

Figure 5.3 illustrates how to characterize the difference between critical reflection and narrative refraction as transitioning from a modern to a postmodern perspective. Ecological learning requires moving back and forth from analytical to narrative

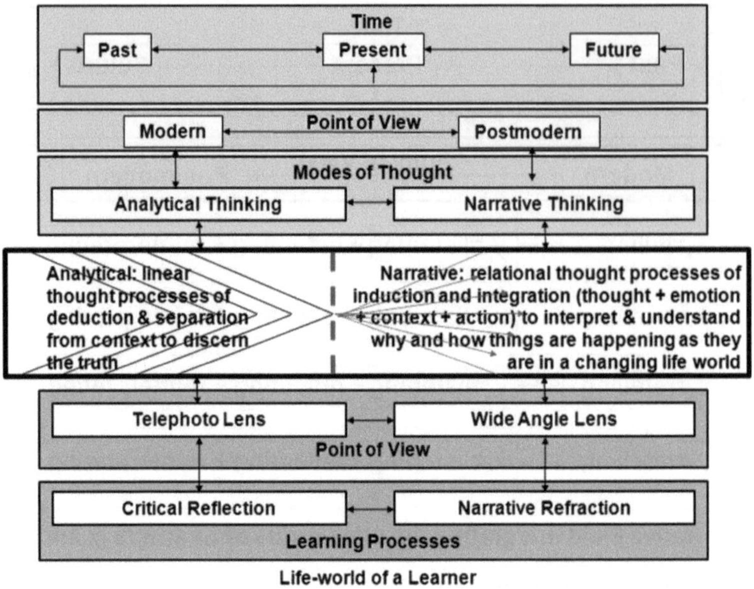

Fig. 5.3 Differentiating and integrating critical reflection and narrative refraction as complementary learning processes (Revision based upon Pfahl 2003 © Nancy Lloyd Pfahl 2009)

thinking, constructing a more holistic perceptual collage from the interaction of paradigmatic and interpretive thought systems in a learner's life-world experience.

We can compare the difference between critical reflection and narrative refraction by considering life-worlds viewed through telephoto and wide-angle lenses, respectively, to interpret life experience. In Fig. 5.3, movement through time encompasses a learning ecology, fluctuating from modern to postmodern points of view, through past, present and future, switching from critical reflection with a telephoto lens to narrative refraction with a wide-angle lens. Thinking deductively (paradigmatically) is analogous to viewing experience through a telephoto lens; thinking inductively (narratively) is analogous to using a wide-angle lens. Understanding the difference between the physical phenomena of reflection (telephoto lens) and refraction (wide angle lens) aids in distinguishing between the learning processes of critical reflection and narrative refraction and their complementary but different learning outcomes. In the physical sciences, reflection is transformation of a figure in which each point is replaced by a point symmetric with respect to a line, merging to a point of light analogous to truth. In critically reflecting upon what we hear, we interpret a text and its meaning as mirror images, an acceptance at face value. The assumption is that what is said and its meaning are the same. Commonly, we expect others to say what they mean, using language in a representational rather than interpretative way. On the other hand, refraction refers to the deflection from a straight path of a ray of light or energy wave as it passes obliquely from one medium into another of different density, as in a wide-angle lens. Various media are analogous to various life experiences.

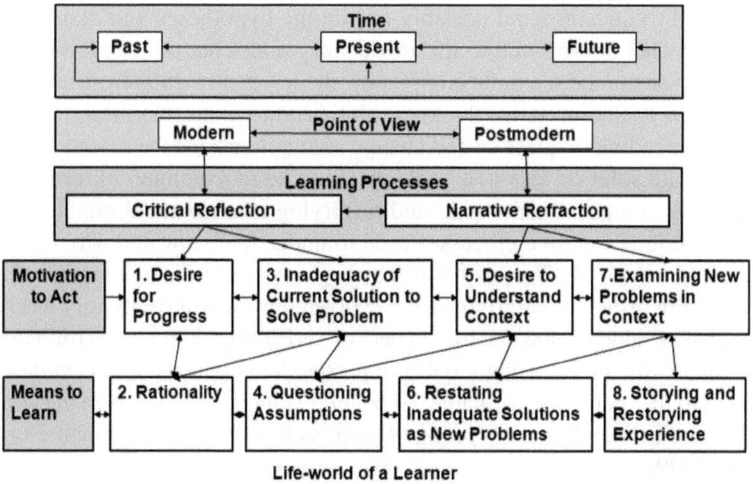

Fig. 5.4 An ecology of learning: Interaction between motivation to act and means to learn within the life-world of a learner (Revision based upon Pfahl 2003 © Nancy Lloyd Pfahl 2009)

Density differences change its speed and bend a ray or wave, changing the form of its image. Similarly, as media of different "densities" bend rays of light or energy waves, stories pass through dissimilar experiences of a teller and a listener to produce different interpretations of meaning in what is heard or seen. Their co-existence does not imply that one interpretation is true and the other is not; they simply inform each other and co-exist with difference. Viewed in this way, narrative processes are refractive rather than reflective, a consequence of the requisite engagement between teller and listener whose bases of life experience differ in "density."

Creating an Ecology of Learning

Making the distinction between critical reflection and narrative refraction creates the capacity to differentiate, name, and link analytical and narrative thought to create an ecology of learning. Figure 5.4 illustrates selected aspects of learning as they relate to modern and postmodern frames of reference.

Consider the example of a research scientist: Beginning with a frame of mind that subscribes to the tenets of modernity, a scientist motivated by a desire to understand a phenomenon (1) relies upon rationality as means to structure and implement a study (2). However, logic does not necessarily lead to understanding the truth about the phenomenon or to an adequate solution for the problem, increasing the scientist's need and motivation to act upon his skepticism to restructure the experiment (3). When logic leads to partial truth and inadequate solutions (3), the scientist is motivated to question and possibly restate the hypotheses and assumptions to understand what contributed to the inadequacy and what to change (4). As new research appears in the scientific community, the researcher shifts from an evaluative point of view to interpretative thinking. Motivated to understand the changed context (5) and needing to question and change assumptions, (4) the researcher restates the inadequate solution as a new problem (6) to be re-examined in relationship to the changing context (7). Storying and restorying to understand implications and meaning are interpretative processes used to understand *how* and *why* from a narrative perspective (8). This scenario that began as traditional scientific research where validity rested in identifying truth evolved into a narrative inquiry where contextual change added value and lifelikeness or verisimilitude-replaced truth (Mishler 1990). Standards for assessing inquiry in postmodern contexts are (1) *authorial*, as attributed to the indeterminate nature of belief; (2) *interpretative*, as in the contextualized nature of belief; and (3) *project-based*, as in the fragmented nature of belief (Bagnall 1999).

Human Learning

What are the commonalities of *human* learning, if not narrative? Human learning integrates interactive simultaneous processes (Jarvis 2006) that are narrative in nature, creating ecology of mind (Bateson 1972). The preceding narrative learning model furthers Jarvis's (2006) interpretation of human learning as an interactive set of simultaneous processes that begin with a socially constructed experience (episode), interpreted as story shaped by narrative processes. Life-world experience is germane to human learning and to narrative, and narrative processes contribute to narrative knowing and shape human learning.

Figure 5.5 illustrates Jarvis's (2006) conception of human learning processes that lead to change (p. 23). His more complicated definition of human learning augments his simple diagram of the process. Human learning is "the combination of processes whereby the whole person – body (genetic, physical and biological) and mind (knowledge, skills, attitudes, values, emotions, beliefs and senses) experiences a social situation, the perceived content of which is then transformed cognitively, emotively or practically (or through any combination) and integrated into the person's individual biography resulting in a changed (or more experienced) person" (Jarvis 2006, p. 13). Action that leads to narrative knowing draws upon a panoply of contributing factors: knowledge, skills, attitudes, values, emotions, beliefs, somatic sensing, intuition, and context.

Following the sequence of Fig. 5.5 in relationship to the preceding narrative model, narration begins with a person in the life-world (1_1) interpreting a socially constructed experience or episode (2). Three simultaneous, cyclical processes advance the learning story: thinking and reflecting (3) to interpret experience through narrative processes of storying and restorying; and examining and interpreting emotion (4)

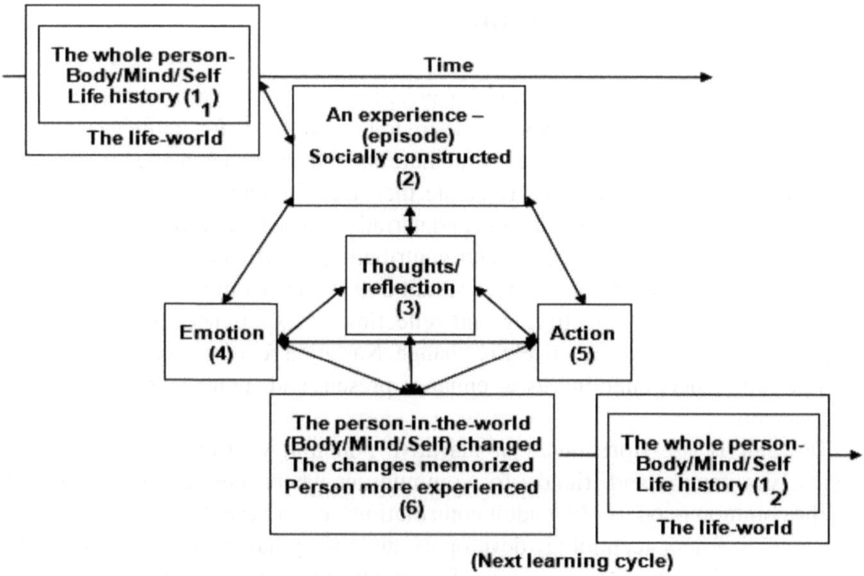

Fig. 5.5 Transformation of a person through learning (Jarvis 2006, p. 23)

associated with experience and made more explicit in story by engaging different factors, including intuition and somatic knowing; and finally taking action (5) that may prompt change that makes a person more experienced (6), as evidenced by future action.

Subsequent stories documenting actions and outcomes in a learner's life history provide evidence of the learner's gaining experience. The stories will show how learning and/or development moved forward constructively or how arrested learning and development resulted in inaction and stagnation. Thereafter, Jarvis's (2006) whole, more experienced learner (1_2) begins another learning cycle or project, employing authorial and interpretative criteria and a postmodern perspective to the learning project in order to learn, develop, and change continually in volatile global, national, and local community contexts.

Jarvis (2006), Bagnall (1999) and other theorists have emphasized connections between learning and change, a relationship implicit in the narrative and human learning models. The models incorporate interaction among the influences of a person's life-world: reflective thought, emotion, and action. They include complementary aspects of how we become more experienced in practice as we narrate experience and couple interpretative texts with narrative analysis to gain a more holistic perspective on life. When a learner transforms experiential content and relates it to personal life history, a more experienced person and expanded life story emerge. This coupling enhances capacity to change by strengthening "individual situational sensitivity, responsiveness, and responsibility" (Bagnall 1999, p. 4).

Responding to Elder Learning Needs

Applying the narrative learning model to elder learning seems particularly appropriate, given the learners' developmental desire to leave a legacy for future generations. Such hope motivates some people to articulate and reflect upon *how* life has unfolded and *why*, in order to create and re-create their realities and identities at different times in their lives. Critical reflection and narrative refraction prompt them to question assumptions that may have been contributing to erroneous or inappropriate actions, attitudes, beliefs, and values (Pfahl 2003). For learning to become developmental, it requires objectifying and reflecting on experience, internalizing its meaning, and acting constructively to change. Narration reorders our understanding of past experience, enabling us to enhance present and future learning response mechanisms.

The elderly are storehouses of narrative potential waiting to be tapped for themselves, family, and friends; for communities where they live and work; and for the common good. If older adult contributions are to benefit the common good, educators, learners, technology developers, and policymakers must recognize that *chronological age* no longer necessarily equates with *functional age*, the capacity to learn, maintain health, remain active, and develop further potential to contribute to society (Butler 2005).

Cultural turbulence and change associated with cyclical life patterns put everyone in a continual state of "*beginnerhood*" (pp. 66–67) that requires continuous action, reflection, and learning in order to survive in today's world of permanent whitewater (Vaill 1996). This instability calls for adaptation and change to address the demographic, social, economic, technological, and political whitewater in the life-worlds of elder learners, educators, and researchers. Collecting and interpreting stories of elder learners' life experiences by using narrative processes of inquiry and analysis can facilitate elder learning and contribute to achieving longevity with capacity. Using the following strategies can facilitate these learning processes:

Foster Lifelong Human Learning and Longevity with Capacity

Re-conceptualizing adult learning as human learning, particularly in the context of lifetime brain plasticity, is a vital consideration for adult educators and longevity professionals. Learning and development, like pedagogy and andragogy, no longer are separate disciplines (Merriam 2001) but elements of a *human* process occurring across the lifespan (Jarvis 2006). One definition of learning is a complex narrative process that integrates contextual, social, rational, emotional, somatic, intuitive, and behavioral phenomena into action-oriented stories that construct and deconstruct identity and reality. Once collected and analyzed thematically and for patterns of action, socially constructed narratives provide multiple perspectives and interpretations of experience, help us learn from difference, and create mutual understanding.

Act with Greater Intentionality

Narration of lived experience to interpret its meaning is a natural entry point to learning; it is an effective strategy that motivates learning, accesses knowing, and weighs possibilities, regardless of age and socio-cultural context (Pfahl and Wiessner 2007; Wiessner and Pfahl 2007). Using narrative processes with greater intentionality naturally induces reinterpretation of the meaning of what has happened. Combining interpretative narrative modes of learning with representational paradigmatic ones is symbiotic. Experimenting with narrative teaching, learning, and research strategies offers rich potential to optimize the way that learners integrate disparate, sometimes conflicting elements of reality to create a more coherent life story. A learning journal can be an effective tool to examine life history and to shape identity (Clark and Rossiter 2008).

Intentional use of narrative reinforces the world's trend toward networked connection. Narrating experience integrates (1) the chaos of our conscious world and (2) subconscious tacit knowledge. Vattimo (1992) links proliferation of mass media to our postmodern condition. Although the linguistic and visual sound bites of text messages, Twitter, and Facebook verge on the point of banality or even meaninglessness for some people, others perceive them as condensed narrative platforms that afford the development of personalized and perpetually evolving narrative language; they create a multidimensional intertwine of social exchange. Over time, space, and context, these linguistic and visual condensations yield personalized iconic styles and become narrative tools by which to connect multiple generations and global participants. It is precisely by maintaining professional awareness of and openness to these newly evolving media among participants of diverse cultural contexts and generations that learning and longevity potential could be furthered.

Support Healthy Living Throughout Life

Knowing that daily life influences mental and physical health and the quality and longevity of our lives, professionals must think creatively about the growing range of older adult lifestyles. Researchers have learned that as we age, active brains are capable of (1) renewing themselves, outdating former assumptions about inevitable brain decline with ageing, and (2) reducing the likelihood of brain debilitation such as what occurs with dementia and Alzheimer's disease (Doige 2007; Just and Varma 2007; Dowling 1998; Kotulak 1996). This growing body of empirical evidence substantiates that physical exercise improves blood flow to our bodies and brains; maintaining lung function ensures that blood carries adequate oxygen to the brain, helping to protect against vascular dementia; continuing education, learning, and mental exercise cause physical changes in the brain, connecting new neural networks and strengthening synapses with continual practice over time; and learning and passion revitalize older adults and help to protect them against degenerative brain diseases such as Alzheimer's. But *how* have healthy elders learned to discipline themselves toward greater capacity in their later years? Narrative inquiry and analysis could answer that question and others.

Elder learners who exhibit intellectual prowess often possess a (1) greater willingness to change and (2) ability to grasp new ideas quickly (Kotulak 1996). Additional attributes characteristic of vital ageing adults include: (3) active engagement in reading, travel, cultural events, education, clubs, and professional associations; (4) lack of chronic diseases; (5) higher standard of living marked by above-average education and income; (6) marriage to an intelligent spouse; (7) brain circuits that allow them to see, think, remember, and act; and (8) satisfaction with their accomplishments (Kotulak 1996). Developmentally, this group of elder learners is well prepared to integrate a lifetime of experience into meaningful narrative legacies.

Reassess Social Economics

How can the elderly serve as valuable resources and add to demographic discourses, including "the prospect of slow growth in productivity, rising public spending [related to healthcare], and labor shortages" (Beck 2009, p. 3)? The growing force of elder learners remains a relatively untapped societal reservoir of wisdom and experience. Desire on the part of many to continue leading active, meaningful lives and the concept of our brain's neuroplasticity reinforces their need for lifelong learning (Hill 2001). What benefits could longevity potential afford to youth, to future evolution of cultural tradition, and to institutional development?

Traditional learning in the East has valued age and experience as a rich social commodity, embedded in communal connectedness and involving mind, body, and spirit. Western tradition, however, has placed less value upon longevity. In Western civilization, there has been a paucity of theological, philosophical, and literary output concerning old age and longevity, perhaps because in the past, old age was attained so infrequently (Butler 2000, p. 23). A literary comparison of Eastern and Western texts could provide a variety of engaging topics for elder learners, educators, and other professionals engaged with longevity-related issues.

Promote Intergenerational Interaction and Learning

Intergenerational communication is akin to communicating cross-culturally and deserves as much attention. Understanding our roots creates feelings of connection that ground us in today's unpredictable world. Although public solidarity requires "bonds between generations" (Attias-Donfut 2000, p. 204), 79% of Americans perceive difficulty in communicating across the generational gap (Pew Research Center 2009). Some postmodern economists argue that it is essential to address problems related to the productivity of *teams* of workers rather than the individual; if that is the case, "the best solution may be to employ a mixture of vigorous young and experienced older workers" (Beck 2009, p. 12). Narrative offers the most accessible means for examining intergenerational collaboration in learning and other environments.

Narratives of experience, narrative inquiry and analysis, and social networking media offer explosive means for connecting across generational, chronological, and spatial barriers. Integrating these resources into innovative intergenerational programs that re-emphasize knowledge, cultural values, and a respect for difference holds potential as means for collaborative learning. Engaging younger and older learners in meaningful dialogue as co-learners and co-teachers creates narratives of shared understanding.

How can new education models network elder learners into youth education programs in order to enrich curricula, increase societal collectivism and motivation, and maximize successes of future generations? Intergenerational interaction is also an important means for (1) expanding adult education goals from development of lifelong learners to facilitation of lifelong community contributors, (2) developing learning content that will contribute to lessening gerontophobia by enhancing elder capacity, and (3) integrating ageing learners into productive community roles.

Conduct Public Dialogues

Professionals have the opportunity to counter stereotypical thinking about ageing through public dialogue and by developing technologies, elder learning programs, and public policies that acknowledge and utilize longevity potential for societal enhancement. Addressing the implications of global demographic change and longevity calls not only for developing and offering courses, but also for public examination of factors that concern the community and influence longevity with capacity.

Consider the following pertinent questions: "Will excessive policy, institutional, or financial power concentrate in the hands of older persons? Will an increase in both the number and percentage of elder adults result in living under a gerontocracy" (Butler 2000, p. 20)? Or, given that the average life expectancy of women is longer than for men, "Will women become the power players in the longevity revolution" (Freidan 1999, p. 237)? Will the longevity revolution complicate issues of resource distribution? "Will elderly medical costs related to incapacity take resources from the young and create intergenerational conflicts" (Butler 2000, p. 20)? How could we tap and utilize the wisdom of elder learners constructively to advance the common good of communities? How could we counter gerontophobia and contribute to preparing younger adults for their elder years? How can we ensure elders equitable integration into the fabric of society? What are our intergenerational responsibilities toward each other? How could we value the wisdom of elders to a greater extent than we now do in the West?

Clearly, adult educators and longevity professionals will play increasingly significant roles in addressing unprecedented change and ensuring "a healthy, vigorous, and educated population to remain both competitive and cooperative" (Butler 2000, p. 21). What is most important for us to remember is that "the full realization of the opportunities resulting from the longevity revolution will depend on many actions that are, in principle, within our control" (Fineberg 2000, p. 288) and that using narrative inquiry and analysis of life stories can play a constructive role in advancing elder learning.

Future Challenges

Narrative shapes life's renewal cycles that alternate between stable *life chapters* and periods of instability – *life transitions* (Hudson 1999 as cited in Butler 2005). Our tumultuous world requires individuals to develop high levels of tolerance for ambiguity and resilience for "continuous reprioritization of the same issues – identity, achievement, intimacy, play, search for meaning, and social compassion" (Hudson 1999, p. 46 as cited in Butler 2005). The importance of narrative learning is substantial, for we sort information by content and by context, and "information that is contextually embedded is easier to learn" (Hill 2001, p. 79).

By its nature, the meaning of narrative lies embedded in context. What can society do to respond to the consequent opportunities and challenges of ambiguity and change, and how can educators assist? Merriam explains: "Adult educators need to become involved in 'building capacities for local groups to engage and confront globalization and its effects at all levels – local, national, and international'" (Schied, Mulenga, & Baptiste 2005, p. 39 as cited in Merriam et al. 2007, p. 15). More intentional use of narrative processes supports such capacity building.

Changing Stagnant Attitudes and Values

What could it mean for our quality of life to become a world of learners with lifelong potential for renewed community contributions after first careers end? Without addressing Western tendencies to (1) put hope to a greater extent in the young, (2) expect the decrement model of ageing, and (3) express surprise at the elderly among us who exhibit exceptional capacity, professionals will not be able to optimize the potential of living longer. The scope of the United States federal legislative initiative "No Child Left Behind" exemplifies the way America, for example, has put its hope for the future in the preparation and achievement of its youngest members of society. But, with demographic shifts in populations across the world, where both the number and percentage of older adults are increasing (Butler 2000) at the same time that the birth rates in most developed countries are declining (United Nations 2009), professionals must rethink education policies and practices to redistribute future hope and educational resources across the lifespan.

Asking Questions, Acting on Findings

How will learning theory, narrative theory, current brain and longevity research, and other factors influence our choices as professionals engaged in active learning and active ageing? Can intentional narrative inquiry further communal learning potential and longevity? How can we respond to longevity challenges and foster concurrent societal benefits? How can we apply new research findings to foster learning that will contribute to longevity *with* capacity? How can education programs and technologies contribute to increasing quality of life and life span of elder learners? To what societal and individual purposes should we use gains in longevity? What are appropriate philosophical, ethical, economic, familial, cultural, and health considerations? What should adult education *become* for elder learners in order to encourage personal fulfillment throughout the lifespan, address implications of the longevity revolution, and develop greater capacity in our elder citizens to contribute to their communities and to the global collective?

Only as we rewrite narrative scripts for the future of elder learning will we facilitate their enactment and discern meaningful answers to these and other emergent questions.

References

Attias-Donfut, C. (2000). Are we moving to a war between the generations? In R. N. Butler & C. Jasmin (Eds.), *Longevity and quality of life: Opportunities and challenges* (pp. 197–213). New York: Kluwer Academic/Plenum Publishers.

Bagnall, R. G. (1999). *Discovering radical contingency: Building a postmodern agenda in adult education*. New York: Peter Lang Publishing Group.

Bateson, G. (1972). *Steps to an ecology of mind*. San Francisco: Chandler Publishing Company.

Bateson, M. C. (2010). *Composing a further life*. New York: Knopf Publishing.

Beck, B. (2009). A slow-burning fire: A special report on ageing populations. *Economist, 391*(8637), 1–16.

Belenky, M. F. & Stanton, A. V. (2000). Inequality, development, and connected knowing. In J. Mezirow & Associates (Eds.), *Learning as transformation: Critical perspectives on a theory in progress* (pp. 71–102). San Francisco: Jossey-Bass.

Boia, L. (2004). *Forever young: A cultural history of longevity from antiquity to the present*. London: BMJ Publishing Group Ltd.

Bruner, J. (1985a). *Actual minds, possible worlds*. Cambridge: Harvard University Press.

Bruner, J. (1985b). Narrative and paradigmatic modes of thought. In E. Eisner (Ed.), *Learning and teaching the ways of knowing* (pp. 97–115). Chicago: The National Society for the Study of Education.

Bruner, J. (1990). *Acts of meaning*. Cambridge: Harvard University Press.

Butler, R. N. (2000). The revolution in longevity. In R. N. Butler & C. Jasmin (Eds.), *Longevity and quality of life: Opportunities and challenges* (pp. 19–23). New York: Kluwer Academic/Plenum Publishers.

Butler, C. B. (2005). Age-related paradigms. In M. A. Wolf (Ed.), *Adulthood: New terrain* (pp. 61–68). San Francisco: Jossey-Bass.

Cell, E. (1984). *Learning to learn from experience*. Albany: State University of New York Press.

Clandinin, M. C., & Connelly, F. M. (1991). Narrative and story in practice and in research. In D. A. Schön (Ed.), *The reflective turn: Case studies in and on educational practice* (pp. 258–282). New York: Teachers College Press.
Clandinin, M. C., & Connelly, F. M. (2000). *Narrative inquiry: Experience and story in qualitative research*. San Francisco: Jossey-Bass.
Clark, M. C., & Rossiter, M. (2008). Narrative learning in adulthood. In S. B. Merriam (Ed.), *Third update on adult learning theory* (pp. 61–70). San Francisco: Jossey-Bass.
Cresswell, J. (1994). *Research design: Qualitative and quantitative approaches*. Thousand Oaks: Sage Publications.
Cross, K. P. (1999). *Learning is about making connections*. Mission Viejo: League for Innovation in the Community College.
Daloz, L. A. (1986). *Effective teaching and mentoring*. San Francisco: Jossey-Bass.
Didion, J. (1979). *The white album*. New York: Farrar, Straus and Giroux.
Doidge, N. (2007). *The brain that changes itself: Stories of personal triumph from the frontiers of brain science*. New York: Penguin Group, Inc.
Dowling, J. E. (1998). *Creating mind: How the brain works*. New York: Norton.
Fineberg, H. V. (2000). Conclusion: Synthesis. In R. N. Butler & C. Jasmin (Eds.), *Longevity and quality of life: Opportunities and challenge* (pp. 287–289). New York: Kluwer Academic/Plenum Publishers.
Freeman, M. (1993). *Rewriting the self: History, memory and narrative*. New York: Routledge.
Freidan, B. (1999). Women in the longevity revolution. In R. N. Butler & C. Jasmin (Eds.), *Longevity and quality of life: Opportunities and challenges* (pp. 235–238). New York: Kluwer Academic/Plenum Publishers.
Gudmundsdottir, S. (1995). The narrative nature of pedagogical knowledge. In H. McEwan & K. Egan (Eds.), *Narrative in teaching, Learning, and research* (pp. 24–38). New York: Teachers College Press.
Hill, L. H. (2001). The brain and consciousness: Sources of information for understanding adult learning. In S. B. Merriam (Ed.), *The new update on adult learning theory* (pp. 73–81). San Francisco: Jossey-Bass.
Jarvis, P. (2006). *Towards a comprehensive theory of human learning*. London: Routledge.
Just, M. A., & Varma, S. (2007). The organization of thinking: What functional brain imaging reveals about the neuroarchitecture of complex cognition. *Cognitive, Affective, & Behavioral Neuroscience, 7*(3), 153–191.
Kasl, E., Marsick, V., & Dechant, K. (1997). Teams as learners: A research-based model of team learning. *The Journal of Applied Behavioral Science, 33*(2), 227–246.
Kegan, R. (1994). *In over our heads: The mental demands of modern life*. Cambridge: Harvard University Press.
Kegan, R. (2000). What "form" transforms? A constructive developmental perspective on transformational learning. In J. Mezirow & Associates (Ed.), *Learning as transformation: Critical perspectives on a theory in progress* (pp. 35–70). San Francisco: Jossey-Bass.
Keller, H., & Werchan, A. (2006). Culture, learning, and adult development. In C. Hoare (Ed.), *Handbook of adult development and learning* (pp. 407–430). New York: Oxford University Press.
Kotulak, R. (1996). *Inside the brain: Revolutionary discoveries of how the brain works*. Kansas City: Andrews McMeel.
Márquez, G. G. (1988). *Love in the time of cholera* (E. Grossman, Trans.). New York: Alfred Knopf.
Marsick, V. J., & Watkins, K. E. (2001). Informal and incidental learning. In S. B. Merriam (Ed.), *The new update on adult learning theory* (pp. 25–34). San Francisco: Jossey-Bass.
Merriam, S. B. (2001). Something old, something new: Adult learning theory for the twenty-first century. In S. B. Merriam (Ed.), *The new update on adult learning theory* (pp. 105–112). San Francisco: Jossey-Bass.
Merriam, S. B., & Clark, M. C. (2006). Learning and development: The connection in adulthood. In C. Hoare (Ed.), *Handbook of adult development and learning* (pp. 27–51). London: Oxford University Press.

Merriam, S. B., & Kim, Y. S. (2008). Non-western perspectives on learning and knowing. In S. B. Merriam (Ed.), *Third update on adult learning theory* (pp. 71–81). San Francisco: Jossey-Bass.

Merriam, S. B., Caffarella, R. S., & Baumgartner, L. M. (2007). *Learning in adulthood: A comprehensive guide* (3rd ed.). San Francisco: Jossey-Bass.

Mishler, E. G. (1986). *Research interviewing: Context and narrative*. Cambridge: Harvard University Press.

Mishler, E. G. (1990). Validation in inquiry-guided research: The role of exemplars in narrative studies. *Harvard Educational Review, 60*, 415–442.

Pew Research Center (2009, June 29). *Growing old in America: Expectations vs. reality: A social & demographic trends report.* http://pewresearch.org/pubs/1269/aging-survey-expectations-versus-reality. Accessed July 3, 2009.

Pfahl, N. L. (2003). *Raising the bar for higher education: Using narrative processes to advance learning and change*. Unpublished dissertation, Columbia University, New York.

Pfahl, N. L., & Wiessner, C. A. (2007). Creating new directions: Drawing on life experiences in community adult education contexts. *Adult Learning, 18*(3 & 4), 9–13.

Piaget, J. (1955). *The child's construction of reality*. London: Routledge.

Polkinghorne, D. (1988). *Narrative knowing and the human sciences*. Albany: State University of New York Press.

Polyani, M. (1966). *The tacit dimension*. Garden City: Doubleday & Company.

Price, J. (1999). In acknowledgment: A review and critique of qualitative research texts. In R. Josselson & A. Lieblich (Eds.), *Making meaning of narrative*. Thousand Oaks: Sage Publications.

Sarbin, T. R. (1986). The narrative as a root metaphor for psychology. In T. R. Sarbin (Ed.), *Narrative psychology: The stories nature of human conduct* (pp. 1–21). Westport: Praeger Publications.

Schaafsma, D. (1993). *Eating on the streets: Teaching literacy in a multicultural society*. Pittsburgh: University of Pittsburgh Press.

Taylor, K., & Lamaroux, A. (2008). Teaching with the brain in mind. In S. B. Merriam (Ed.), *Third update on adult learning theory* (pp. 49–59). San Francisco: Jossey-Bass.

United Nations Department of Economic and Social Affairs. (2009). *World population prospects 2004: Analytical report* (Population Studies No. 246). http://un.orglesa/population/publications/wppp2003_VOL_3.pdf. Accessed February 11, 2009.

Vaill, P. B. (1996). *Learning as a way of being: Strategies for surviving in a world of permanent whitewater*. San Francisco: Jossey-Bass.

Vattimo, G. (1992). *The transparent society* (D. Webb, Trans.). Baltimore: The Johns Hopkins University Press.

Wiessner, C. A., & Pfahl, N. L. (2007). Choosing different lenses: Using storytelling as a narrative technique to promote knowledge construction and learning in adults. *The Journal of Continuing Higher Education, 55*(1), 27–37.

Merriam, S. B., & Kim, Y. S. (2008). Non-western perspectives on learning and knowing. In S. B. Merriam (Ed.), *Third update on adult learning theory* (pp. [illegible]). San Francisco: Jossey-Bass.

Merriam, S. B., Caffarella, R. S., & Baumgartner, L. M. (2007). *Learning in adulthood: A comprehensive guide* (3rd ed.). San Francisco: Jossey-Bass.

Mishler, E. G. (1986). *Research interviewing: Context and narrative*. Cambridge: Harvard University Press.

[illegible]

Chapter 6
Toward Critical Narrativity: Stories of Ageing in Contemporary Social Policy*

Simon Biggs

Introduction

Social Policy as Narrative

How does social policy, and the stories it tells, influence the spaces in which we might grow old? There can be little doubt that narrativity, the use of a "story" metaphor, both as a research technique (Holstein and Gubrium 2000; Kenyon et al. 1999) and as a technique for personal self-construction (McAdams 1993; McLeod 1997), is becoming increasingly popular both within and beyond social gerontology. Part of the attractiveness of thinking in terms of stories is the opening of a critical space between description and intention. It makes it much easier to sidestep social determinacy and take a stance toward positions that might otherwise present themselves as the only possible reality. This does not mean that such narratives should be taken lightly, however, especially when they exist in the public sphere of social policy. They have the power, it is argued, to shape behavior and expectation, and thus, considerable political energy is invested in their promotion and maintenance.

In the last 20 years, western social policy has seen significant shifts in its ideological base. There has been a move away from welfarism, which was found in its classic form in the UK, Australia, and New Zealand, toward market-based "mixed economies" of social care.

Rationales and mechanisms were adopted from US and Canadian systems, which were themselves undergoing an intensification of these same trends. Methods such

* Previously published in *Journal of Aging Studies* (2001), *15*: 303–316.

S. Biggs (✉)
School of Social and Political Sciences, University of Melbourne,
Melbourne, VIC, Australia
e-mail: biggss@unimelb.edu.au

G.M. Boulton-Lewis and M. Tam (eds.), *Active Ageing, Active Learning: Issues and Challenges*, Education in the Asia-Pacific Region: Issues, Concerns and Prospects 15,
DOI 10.1007/978-94-007-2111-1_6, © Springer Science+Business Media B.V. 2012

as case-management were used, to "marketize" the unitary welfare state on the one hand, and manage the fragmentation of services and resources on the other. If such methods transform and mediate economic relations, they also influence the perception helping professionals and clients of services have of themselves. They become, to use a Foucaultian term, technologies of the self (Biggs and Powell 2000).

In each of the countries mentioned above, older people are the majority group using health and social care services (Phillipson 1998). It would be peculiar, then, if changes in public policy had not been accompanied by changing narratives of old age. The character, significance, and consequences of such narratives which it is argued make a significant contribution to what Holstein and Gubrium (2000) have referred to as "selves we live by," is the subject of this chapter. Particular attention will be paid to the turn, seemingly away from market ideology toward a social-democratic "third way" approach to social issues. This turn will be interrogated in terms of its ideological and material determinants, its focus and what it fails to address, and its consequences for the construction of an ageing identity under contemporary conditions.

Why Is Social Policy Important?

Social policy is not simply a governing body's concerned response to a particular problem or social ill that can then be remedied, however much professional politicians may wish, and sometimes believe this to be the case (Decalmer and Glendenning 1997). This interpretation positions policy making as a benign rescuer from problems that blow in like a natural disaster or are uncovered by the forward March of progress. It is a story itself about causality and appropriateness of response.

Writers such as Bourdieu (2000) and Foucault (1980) have made it much harder to avoid the fact that policies not only respond to social ills, they also consecrate them. They contribute to the constellation of ideas and evidence that create the problem itself. Creation is being used in at least two senses here: as a contribution toward the material conditions, either through action or inaction, that increases the likelihood that a certain social ill will occur; and in the sense that through the agency of social policy formation, certain issues are legitimized. They are shaped and made visible in particular ways.

For the helping professional, this often means that policy is permissive of certain activities and prohibitive of others. This is especially true tor public sector and related professionals who are close to and by degrees dependent upon the political executive. At the most fundamental level, policy makes material resources available to pursue those activities. From an institutional point of view, it allows certain social issues to be "seen," to be recognized and therefore addressed.

However, policy can also do more than that in furnishing a vision or series of visions of experience, such as later life, which legitimize a place in which social subjects are able to form publicly acceptable identities. Such frameworks, according to Charles Taylor (1989) "Provide the background, explicit or implicit, for our moral judgments, intuitions or responses . . . My identity . . . is the horizon within which I am capable of making a stand" (p. 26).

For Taylor, the possibility of making a moral stand is intimately tied up with the surrounding social framework, and becomes an amalgam of self-directed invention and the degree to which circumstances facilitate the expression of an identity acceptable to one's moral self. Can one, in other words, take a stand toward something and how easy or difficult is that possibility made? In order to take a stand, one has to be able to identify the "something," and have the resources to stand up to or for it.

The interrogation of policy as a contradictory space, both a Foucaultian determinant of legitimizing discourse and as one of Taylor's sites that can enable critical alternatives to emerge, introduces us to a continuum along which the very possibility of being able to conceive an alternative state of affairs is in itself problematic. It links formal policy positions to personal experience in a way that emphasizes the likelihood of critical awareness. At first (or perhaps more accurately when starting from a singularly bleak and repressive point), an existing state of affairs might be unquestioningly accepted. A little further along the continuum, it may be experienced as a troubling sense of "not-rightness" that cannot easily be put into words, but which nevertheless challenges, through intuitions however slight, the status quo. We are dealing in the degree to which words can be found and whether a sense of resistance can make the leap from private, inner discourse to a public statement of belief and agency. It is as if particular narratives invite a series of steps from an inability to conceive of an alternative state of affairs or even open oneself to the intuition that something may not be quite right to the articulation of resistance and more advanced still, a vision of a different possibility. This possibility of authenticity (as in when the interior life can find expression through the social sphere rather than the latter simply being internalized as social conformity; when narratives engage the imagination through living more fully; as, in other words, a political act), I have begun to examine elsewhere (Biggs 1999a, b). Here, I want to explore in more detail the possibility of influencing our imaginations through social policy, which is another way of saying political persuasion.

The imagination is not, in this sense, an entirely interior phenomenon. It is subject to a good story being told. It needs grounding in an externally legitimated narrative process. It needs to be engaged.

From Structured Dependency to Age as Opportunity

I would like to use the social-democratic turn in UK social policy as a case example. This turn broadly follows the transition from a virtual hegemony of free-market policies as applied to the welfare of older people that followed the Thatcher/Reagan years. A turn toward something else, sometimes referred to as a "third way," emerging under Clinton, Blair, and Schroeder administrations in the US and parts of Europe. In terms of social policy, this third way can be thought of as an attempt to fashion a different position from those constituted by the traditional welfare state on the one hand, and an unbridled marketplace on the other. The third way, in so far as it exists, has drawn both on Communitarian thinking from the United States and European Policies for Social Inclusion (Byrne 1999; Jordan 1996). Its ideological origins and implications for older people will be elaborated shortly. However, it is first necessary to situate these developments in their historical context.

Structured Dependency in the Welfare State and the Market

Prior to the social-democratic turn in western politics, a narrative held sway that was characterized by increasing dependency as adults aged. This held true, at least in social policy thinking as a substrate of both welfarism and market approaches. It was typical of an unreflective perspective on adult ageing, which, as Lynott and Lynott (1996) have pointed out, left little room for critical analysis and the development of an alternative story line. It is a perspective that has been criticized by a number of writers, such as Estes (1979, 1993) and Minkler and Estes (1998) in the US, and Phillipson (1982, 1998), Townsend (1981, 1986), and Walker (1986, 1996) in the UK, who have viewed the social construction of ageing through the lens of political economy.

The general consensus to be found within a political economy approach states that dependence in later life is not an inevitable and biologically determined "fact of life," but is artificially created by a number of economic mechanisms. The emphasis given to each mechanism varies from writer to writer and includes: the forced expulsion of older people from the workforce, the growth and self-promotion of professional interests, the manipulation of vulnerable older people as if they were commodities in a welfare market and a marginalization of later life concerns. These various forms of ageist oppression are held together, it is argued, on a widely held but at root economically determined, perception of older people as unproductive and a burden on society as a whole.

This view is substantiated, even at the birth of the British welfare state, in William Beveridge's statement that it might be "dangerous to be in any way lavish to old age" until the needs of other parts of the population have been met. As recently as 1988, it has not been unusual to find statements such as the following, taken from an annual review of government statistics.

"Although the size of the dependent population in 2025 will not be much higher than it was in 1971, its composition will be different in that there will be far less children and many more elderly people, so reducing the demand for education, but increasing the burden on health services" (Social Trends 1988).

Accordingly, it can be surmised that policy makers viewed older adults as both burdensome and ineducable. If education and health services are perceived to be an economic investment in the future or existing workforce, then it is unsurprising that, as a political economy critique would predict, older people are both denied them and stigmatized into the bargain.

In so far as older people were allowed a space in which to make their stand, this was located within the traditional welfare state and most notably under the auspices of health, pensions, and social care policy. Use it or resist it, or do the two together, the welfare state, with all its faults, provided a socially legitimate locus for late life concerns.

While the marketization of welfare in the 1980s and 1990s treated the users of services as consumers with certain rights, a combination of factors eroded this space, including the removal of tree services, the transfer of responsibilities onto informal care and an eclipsing of requirements specific to older people within a generic, consumerist orientation. In other words, the new market appeared not to replace the traditional welfare state with a viable alternative space in which to develop a positive ageing identity, other than as an ageless consumer or depending upon mental capacity, as a commodity (Biggs and Powell 2000; Phillipson and Biggs 1998). Neither of these positions recognize the particular opportunities associated with later life and the possibility of successful ageing (Baltes and Baltes 1990; Rowe and Kahn 1998) nor do they address the particular risks that later life can bring with it (other than in the sense that these positions constitute significant risks in themselves).

The vision of the older person as a consumer was, of course, not without its ideological and material correlates. The growth of a "gray market" and distinctive lifestyles amongst affluent older people has been noted on both sides of the Atlantic (Featherstone and Hepworth 1982; Gilleard 1996; S. Katz, personal communication, 2000; Sawchuk 1995). Further, these changes have given rise to a view associated with the postmodernization of social theory, that under certain circumstances, older people might free themselves not only of the social but also the bodily constraints of growing old (Featherstone and Hepworth 1995). This perspective has been critiqued elsewhere (Biggs 1997, 1999b; Phillipson 1998), however. It also resonates with and, to an extent, underpins, "third way" notions of older people. Here, elders are seen as part of the citizenry who are both able to choose certain "leisured" lifestyles and have the capacity to participate much more effectively in a variety of social arenas than was previously thought possible. As such, it appeared to point to a new space or series of spaces, within which ageing identities could take shape. The older person, under the gaze of social policy analysis, was becoming not simply a consumer but an autonomous participant in civil society.

A Third Way for the Third Age

In the new millennium, the British Government has embarked upon a large, if not to say baffling, array of initiatives to promote positive ageing. It is at first sight puzzling why so much energy is being put into something that is not, in the UK context, an obvious vote winner. Indeed, general public awareness of the initiatives themselves appears to be low (Employers Forum on Age 2000). These initiatives, which will be outlined later in this chapter, constitute a significant attempt to engineer a new identity for British elders and counteract ones based on decrement and disengagement. It constitutes a sharp break with previous policies toward older people and is seductive for social gerontologists in so far as it seems to have learned many of the lessons preached about ageism, structured dependency, and passivity in later life.

In order to understand the overt motivation for such an abrupt policy turn, it is necessary to place these new policies on ageing within the context of the wider analysis and concerns of the social-democratic project.

Blairite social policy rests on the notion that the 1997 Labour Government inherited a social fabric that had been placed under severe strain, following almost two decades of unbridled market economics. There were resulting problems of social exclusion, with significant sections of the population being or in danger of becoming disaffected and ceasing to identify with the British State as a cohesive focus for national identity.

Thus, in 1997, shortly after coming to power, Blair made the following continent on the steps of a public housing project: "Behind the statistics lie households where three generations have never had a job. There are estates where the biggest employer is the drugs industry (sic), where all that is left of the high hopes of the post-war planners is derelict concrete. Behind the statistics are people who have lost hope, trapped in fatalism" (Social Exclusion Unit website 2.6.1997).

In the years following the Second World War, British National identity had become closely associated with the welfare state. The welfare state functioned, then, not simply as a source of material support to the most vulnerable and excluded. It also provided an imaginative focus, as an indicator, of a caring society and of national coherence and inclusiveness. Neo-Thatcherite policies had, however, characterized welfarism as a source of social dependency and a drain on an enterprise culture (Walker 1995).

If the Neo-Thatcherite remedy for social problems had been almost Foucaultian in its inspiration, increasingly putting in place mechanisms of surveillance to monitor and control disaffected or vulnerable adults, including older people and their caretakers (Biggs and Powell 2000; Powell and Biggs 2000), the social-democratic response was arguably Gramscian. Disaffected groups should be encouraged to identify once more with an inclusive national project and put aside their conflicts of interest. The policy solution to the diagnosis of social exclusion would therefore be to bring as many groups as possible to identify with the national and local state, and that included older people.

Blair continues, "The basis of this modern civic society is an ethic of mutual responsibility and duty. It is something for something, a society where we play by the rules. You only take out if you put in. That's the bargain" (Social Exclusion Unit, 2.6.97).

Further, "The most meaningful stake anyone can have in society is the ability to earn a living and support a family" (Blair 1996, p. 34).

Thus, the policy aims of this period included undoing the fragmentation caused by radical market policies, while learning from them by not wishing to directly remedy social problems. A focus on family obligation and the value of work might not have been the most auspicious start for an antiageist policy, especially as Blair's (1996) personal manifesto was entitled: "New Britain: My vision of a young country."

The role of government was not, then, to increase expenditure on pensions and services, but to create spaces in which civil society can take a certain shape and that shape depended on the value of work and of the family. Neither of these spaces – the workplace and family life – were necessarily amenable to older people who were excluded from the former and often entrapped by the latter (Phillipson 1998).

However, a heady mixture of an increased awareness of ageism as a form of social exclusion and postmodern late-lifestyleism leads to an attempt to reinvent adult ageing: from being a problem of burden to an age of opportunity. Blair again states, "My vision is for a society in which older people are given more say in how services are run . . . We need to value and celebrate older people for the experience they bring and the active contribution they can make. They are an essential part of the Britain I want to build" (Blair 1996).

Social-Democratic Initiatives on Ageing

What Are the Initiatives?

High-level Government interest in older people has led to a series of initiatives in a variety of arms of government, including the following:

- "Better Government for Older People" (www.bettergovernment for olderpeople.gov.uk). Addressing Public Services and set up in 1998 to "improve public services for older people by better meeting their needs, listening to their views and encouraging and recognizing their contribution" (All Our Futures 2000, pp. a4–b10). Better Government for Older People has been responsible for a large number of partnerships between older people's representatives and local government. It has no defined age group as its target, however, a view has begun to emerge that "50 plus" is important "in breaking down traditional barriers of ageism and the state retirement age, as well as drawing younger people into debate and strategies for an ageing population" (Strategem 2000, p. 2).
- In the National Health Service (NHS), a National Service Framework (NHF), setting out standards and best practice in certain key areas has been created to address the needs of older people (www.doh.gov·uk/nsf). It is stated in The NHS Plan (2000) that "The NSF will ensure that ageism is not tolerated in the NHS, with the elimination of any arbitrary policies based on age alone" (p. 15.6). This is in part a response to a series of campaigns led by the charity Age Concern England whose report: "Turning Your Back on Us: Older People and the NHS" attacks the government claim of "equal treatment for all" citing Gallop surveys on refusals of treatments, lower quality treatment, and with age-related formal and informal "cutoffs" for receipt of treatment.

- On the Employment issues, the relevant department has published: "Age Diversity in Employment" (June 1999) (www.dfee.gov.uk/age diversity/code), which includes a Code of Practice, guidance, and case studies. Emphasis has been placed on age discrimination across the life course, which can be remedied by merit-based decision taking and access to training. This document broadly follows the position of the Employers Forum on Age (2000) (www.efa.ogr.uk/ace/efa) in aiming to remove barriers to achieving "an age-balanced work-force" and promote the "business benefits of employing a mixed age workforce." There is, however, a significant exception to the document and the views of the EFA, Age Concern, and Better Government for Older People in so far as legislation to prohibit age discrimination has not, at the time of writing, been proposed.
- Finally, in the area of *Consumption*, the "Foresight" initiative sponsored by the Department of Trade and Industry has identified older people as a significant market opportunity for the new millennium. In its own words, "Foresight brings together the voices of business, government, the sciencebase and others to identify the threats and opportunities that we are likely to face over the next 10–20 years" (2000, p. i).

The Ageing Population Panel (April 1999) (www.foresight.gov.uk) notes that, "The reshaping of the age pyramid will reach into all corners of society. It offers fresh opportunities for businesses large and small … There will be major international opportunities, especially in countries … which experienced sustained and intense baby booms after the war … If British business is to remain competitive, employers will need to make better use of older people in the workforce. For its part, Government will need to ensure that the financing of pensions does not impose an unsustainable tax burden and that individuals can provide for themselves in old age" (2000, p. 4). Thus, in a variety of ways, an ageing population is being redefined as a social, political, and economic opportunity.

Joining Up the Dots

A key aim of social-democratic policy has been to ensure that broad social initiatives do not become enmired in the competing priorities of particular government departments. To this end, an unprecedented step was taken in creating mechanisms at the center of government to progress policy on ageing. This has included an *Inter-Ministerial Group on Older People* reporting to the Prime Minister's own Cabinet Office. It has also included creating a *Cabinet Champion for Older People* in Alistair Darling, also Secretary of State for Social Security. Initially, a keynote strategic document was produced, entitled: "Building A Better Britain for Older People" (Nov 1998) (www.dss.gov.uk/hq/pubs/older/html/index.htm) and quaintly referred to as B.BOP. B.BOP states that the work of helping people to continue leading an "active, independent and secure life" … "is likely to focus on ways that of improving the quality of life of older people, by making it easier for them to stay active for longer in their communities, either through employment or volunteering" ... plus ... "To end age discrimination in the workforce" and maintain "active lives through mentoring, volunteering and lifelong learning" (1998, pp. 4 and 6). This sentiment has been followed through in a series of further documents, culminating in a summarizing policy report: "Winning the Generation Game" (Policy Innovation Unit 2000) (www.cabinetoffice.gov.uk/innovation/2000/winning/active/foreward.htm). The Employers' Forum on Ageing has indicated that the recommendations made in this report "will have an influence across Government and the agenda for the rest of 2000 and beyond" (EFA webpage 2000).

The Prime Minister's Forward to the report states that "One of the most important tasks for twenty-first century Britain is to unlock the talents and potential of all its citizens. Everybody has a valuable contribution to make, throughout their lives. Unless we encourage older people to remain actively engaged in socially valued activity, whether paid or unpaid, everybody in Britain will miss out on the benefits of their experience and social commitment" (Policy Innovation Unit webpage 2000, p. 1).

It thus picks up on the themes of exclusion and opportunity that are key to the policy initiative on positive ageing; however, these opportunities are interpreted in a particular way, and the space within which older people might make their stand is limited in its scope.

The report consolidates a number of themes and focuses the policy concern such that it is "about people between 50 and State Pension Age and their engagement in economic and community activity." Four key areas for further action include:

- Changing the culture: "to raise expectations of older people and stop making judgements based on their age rather than their true value and potential'.
- Enabling over 50s to stay in work: increased work flexibility, skill development, and reduced "perverse incentives" – which the report interprets as the "distortions" of early retirement and the cost of funding persons thereby retired.
- Helping displaced workers to re-enter work, job-seeking support, and changing the attitudes of benefit staff.
- Helping older people make use of their skills and experience for the benefit of the wider community. This highlights volunteering as "making use of the experience and availability" of retired people.

So where does this leave us? For older people, a narrative is emerging of social value through work or near-work situations. If you are active, volunteering and mentoring are identified as legitimized fields of social inclusion, plus the possibility of an extended period of formal work. This fits nicely with policy anxiety about a falling labor force. If you are in some way incapacitated, then your problems are interpreted primarily as problems of access and of changing the attitudes of health and social care staff.

This is a tremendous move away from a narrative of dependency and evidences a progressive refinement of the question of ageing and the nature of the "opportunity" it presents. We are told a story of autonomous older people, actively involved in their communities, achieving joy through the return of work and voluntary activities.

It also appears that later life is being defined as a relatively homogeneous part of the life course, beginning at approximately age 50. Work-like activities are presented as a sort of social therapy that capitalizes on postmodern ageing and simultaneously draws older people back into the social mainstream. Another marginalized group is saved!

It Is Still the Economy, Stupid

Following the social policy narrative across departments of Government, there appears to be considerable achievement in replacing a story of decline in later life with one that places successful ageing and antiageism firmly on the agenda. As such, the UK experience parallels a dense mix of positive antiageist rhetoric and anti-dependency programming that is becoming a characteristic of policy across the western world (S. Katz, personal communication, 2000). This turn in the tale is particularly seductive for social gerontology as it appears to be in close agreement with much of what gerontologists have been saying. Increased social expectations of older people allow a new series of places on which to build an ageing identity. Attempts at joined-upness in the Government executive complement the complexity of late-life issues. Recognition is made that the attitudes and aspirations of some sectors of the older population are changing radically (Boaz and Hayden) and that this is true both in terms of social structuration (Phillipson 1998) and in terms of personal identity (Biggs 1999b).

However, on closer inspection, the narrative of ageing that emerges as a result of policy priorities is significantly limited in its scope. It is also increasingly unclear whether the particular interpretations of success are ones that dovetail with the material requirements of older adults or with the demands of other groups within advanced capitalism and high modernity.

For example, while statements from the Better Government for Older People agenda are driven by older people's groups and organizations, and tend to emphasize the need for fiscal security through state pensions and improved services, other groups such as Foresight focus on financial autonomy. When one looks at the rationale behind the "summarizing document" *Winning the Generation Game*, the economic reasoning behind positive ageing policies becomes quite clear. Here, the need for changing lifestyles in later life is closely linked to the fiscal implications of an ageing population.

- By 2031, 41% of our country will be over 50, 23% over retirement age and 6% over 80.
- With present employment rates, there will be one million more over 50s not working by 2020 because of the growth of the older population.
- There will be two million fewer working age people under 50 and two million more over 50 – a shift equivalent to nearly 10% of the total working population.
- Most people leaving work have not done so voluntarily, almost half who do are dependent on state benefits and often experience disillusionment and exclusion.

- Drop in work rates amongst under 50s since 1979 – cost per annum. £16 billion in lost gross domestic product and £3–5 billion in benefits and lost taxes (PDU 2000, p. 2.2).

There is, in other words, concern that there will be too few workers around to meet the needs of capital and too many ex-workers demanding benefits if current social attitudes prevail. The solution, the "opportunity" therefore lies in redefining later life by encouraging work (thus, solving the employment shortfall) and discouraging retirement that is not resourced by elders on an individual and privatized basis (thus, reducing demand on the benefits system). Active ageing defined as work and volunteering (unpaid work) balances the books nicely. Each arm of Government follows the same narrative, adapted to local circumstances. Thus, Local Government and Public Service see elders as engaged in participation and service partnership. For the Department of Social Security, a preoccupation with lost taxes and costs of benefits makes work the answer. For Trade and Industry, older people are self-sufficient consumers in a new "gray" market.

If narratives of ageing are based on work or work-like activities, certain problems arise. Autonomy is by no means the same as freedom under these conditions, however much it masquerades as such. First, there is a tendency to confuse social inclusion and work or community activity that restricts visibility of other forms of contribution that do not rely upon conformity to a work ethic for their social value. Unseen activities such as caretaking activities and delegitimized activities such as political dissidence do not seem to appear on this agenda. Second, there is confusion, at least in UK policy, over the role of education. While one policy document, *Life Begins at 50* (2000), places it with "lifelong learning and leisure," the Department of Employment and Education within whose field of operations one might reasonably expect it to appear has lost lifelong learning through a preoccupation with children's education and vocational reskilling. Third, if volunteering and participation become a sort of social therapy rather than genuinely inclusive activities (Carter and Beresford 2000), they become just as much a "playpen for the old" as have other forms of "retirement community" activity (Kuhn 1977). Such activities contribute to the "storying" of older people as included through "participation" rather than through increased provision, and to say that participation has a positive health and social outcome is not the same as giving a specific response to a specific service requirement.

Like the postmodern reshaping of ageing as a matter of midlife styles (Featherstone and Hepworth 1982), this policy narrative solves the problem of ageing by assuming that older people are the same as everyone else. In terms of equity, this makes sense if it encourages the removal of barriers to equal treatment. However, it may be inaccurate to characterize older people as having the same abilities (to do the same jobs as younger adults) and needs (without special requirements because of disabilities associated with age) as other sections of the population. There is an astonishing absence of diversity in policies that assume that everyone from a white male in his fifties to a black woman in her nineties has the same personal and social priorities. Indeed, the one area where work and work-related activities do hold out the possibility of commonality, in terms of solidarity across the generations around the terms and conditions of work and the responsibilities of employers, is remarkable by its absence. Interpretations of the life tasks of maturity that emphasize other potentialities surrounding ageing – spirituality (Howse 1999), gero-transcendence (Tornstam 1996), "the well-earned rest" and contemplation through "coming to terms with oneself" – may not be compatible with an active/positive narrative of productive ageing. There are thus at least two problems with building a policy about ageing on similarity in the way described above. On the one hand, it only focuses on the equal right to compete for work, without acknowledging the common interests of workers across generations, and on the other, it ignores any form of diversity in ageing priorities that do not fit the work-related pattern as defined by the dominant discourse.

In summary, it is possible to pose and work toward certain answers to the following questions about the social-democratic turn in ageing policy.

It is possible to say the following on how facilitative the policy environment is, and the "internal logic" of the story being told there. At first sight, "new ageing" policies appear to be highly facilitative. They challenge ageism, particularly as it affects access to work and services. They recognize a greater flexibility in "postmodern" lifestyles, income, and potential in later life. They highlight the importance of social inclusion and autonomy for older people, and so long as one stays within that thinking loop, the policy hangs together. However, such internal coherence requires a certain ignorance of social inequality and diversity of desire amongst older people. It creates a narrative that is facilitative for older people with the ability to finance a "midlife style" and want, or have the physical or mental capacity, to participate in existing social institutions. It encourages inclusion of a type that privileges work and activities that take a work-like form. As a place in which to stand and build an ageing identity, this story of late-life development is, however, lacking. It lacks critical edge, and at root it has little place for dissident or alternative pathways for self and social development other than through work.

The surface logic of the story corresponds only tangentially with the deeper or wider circumstances of economic priorities, driven by a perceived need to drive down support to older persons and create a reserve pool of labor. Moreover, older people should be grateful for this "opportunity" because it cements them into a situation in which they will not be excluded from the mainstream.

On Critical Narrativity

As the argument in this paper has developed, narrativity has emerged both as a content issue, narratives being told to us about later life, and as a technique for interrogating that content in terms of its surface appearance and underlying trajectory. As such, a critical narrativity, as explored in this paper, evokes Cole's (1992) observation that there is an implied dualism in the way in which western societies conceptualize ageing. Ageing is, then, split into positive and negative attributes that are separated either between population groups, or, as in the present case, different levels of rhetoric. At the beginning of this paper, it was observed that a narrative approach makes it much easier to sidestep social determinacy and take a stance toward positions that might otherwise present themselves as the only possible reality. While this property may account for the popularity of narrativity in so far as it is perceived as emphasizing human agency, it also has a shadow side. The gap between material realities and the story told can lead to a number of perversions, which in policy terms may allow the sidestepping of social contradictions, the doing of one thing while discoursing another, and the possibility of writing a story, for social policy purposes with internal coherence, which only makes sense so long as you do not step outside of it. This, however, is not to denigrate the role of the imaginative in policy space. Rather, the question becomes how far a narrative allows a stand to be taken and how convincing is the narrative in inviting a new terrain for struggle.

There are a number of issues that then force themselves upon a critical social gerontology. Firstly, what forms of ageing are legitimated and delegitimized by a particular narrative. Secondly, how far alternative narrative positions correspond to the social and political experience of older people. Thirdly, whether an inauthentic political initiative, in the sense that a stated intention masks a different and potentially inimicable underlying trajectory, can nevertheless contribute to social spaces in which a more authentic and thereby fulfilling ageing can be achieved.

The development of policy narratives that appear simultaneously to critically engage ageism, yet present alternative stories that are in themselves restrictive and prey to interests that are inimicable to those of older people, appears to be an international phenomenon. It is in many ways a more complex phenomenon than narratives of decline and dependency. The critical space that narrativity can open between rhetoric and experience allows an interrogation of these trends. We are being told a tale, but we do not necessarily have to believe it.

References

Age Concern England. (2000). *Turning your back on us: Older people and the NHS*. London: ACE.

Baltes, P., & Baltes, M. (1990). *Successful ageing: Perspectives from the behavioral sciences*. New York: Cambridge University Press.

Better Government for Older People. (2000). *All our futures. Pts: (a) All our futures. (b) Making a difference. (c)Our present for the future*. Wolverhampton: BGOP.

Biggs, S. (1997). Choosing not to be old? *Ageing & Society, 17*, 553–570.

Biggs, S. (1999a). The blurring of the life course: Narrative, memory and the question of authenticity. *Journal of Aging and Identity, 44*, 209–221.

Biggs, S. (1999b). *The mature imagination*. Buckingham: Open University Press.

Biggs, S., & Powell, J. (2000). A Foucauldian analysis of old age and the power of social welfare. *Journal of Aging & Social Policy, 8*, 43–49.

Blair, T. (1996). *New Britain: My vision for a young country*. London: Fourth Estate.

Bourdieu, P. (2000). *Pascalian meditations*. Cambridge: Polity.

Byrne, P. (1999). *Social exclusion*. Buckingham: Open University Press.

Carter, T., & Beresford, P. (2000). *Age and change: Models of involvement for older people*. New York: JRF.

Cole, T. (1992). *The journey of life*. New York: Cambridge University Press.
Decalmer, P., & Glendenning, F. (1997). *The mistreatment of older people*. London: Sage.
EFA webpage (2000) (www.efa-online.org)
Employers Forum on Age (2000) (www.efa.ogr.uk/ace/efa)
Estes, C. (1979). *The aging enterprise*. San Francisco: Jossey-Bass.
Estes, C. (1993). The aging enterprise re-visited. *The Gerontologist, 33*(3), 292–298.
Featherstone, M., & Hepworth, M. (1982). Ageing and inequality; Consumer culture and the new middle age. In D. Robbins (Ed.), *Rethinking inequality* (pp. 97–126). London: Gower.
Featherstone, M., & Hepworth, M. (1995). Images of positive ageing. In M. Featherstone & A. Wernick (Eds.), *Images of ageing* (pp. 29–47). London: Routledge.
Foucault, M. (1980). *Power/knowledge*. London: Harvester.
Gilleard, C. (1996). Consumption and identity in later life. *Ageing & Society, 16*, 489–498.
Holstein, J., & Gubrium, J. (2000). *The self we live by*. New York: Oxford University Press.
Howse, K. (1999). *Religion, spirituality and older people*. London: CPA.
Jordan, B. (1996). *A theory of poverty and social exclusion*. Cambridge: Polity.
Kenyon, G., Ruth, J., & Mader, W. (1999). Elements of a narrative gerontology. In V. Bengtson & K. Schaie (Eds.), *Handbook of theories of aging* (pp. 40–58). New York: Springer.
Kuhn, T.S. (1977). *The Essential Tension: Selected Studies in Scientific Tradition and Change*. Chicago and London: University of Chicago Press.
Lynott, R., & Lynott, P. (1996). Tracing the course of theoretical development in the sociology of aging. *The Gerontologist, 36*(6), 749–760.
McAdams, D. (1993). *The stories we live by*. New York: Morrow.
McLeod, J. (1997). *Narrative and psychotherapy*. London: Sage.
Minkler, M., & Estes, C. (1998). *Critical gerontology; Perspectives from political and moral economy*. New York: Baywood.
PDU (2000) – a typo, should be PIU (Policy Innovation Unit, 2000) (www.cabinetoffice.gov.uk/innovation/2000/winning/active/foreward.htm)
Phillipson, C. (1982). *Capitalism and the construction of old age*. London: Macmillan.
Phillipson, C. (1998). *Reconstructing old age*. London: Sage.
Phillipson, C., & Biggs, S. (1998). Modernity and identity: Themes and perspectives in the study of older adults. *Journal of Aging and Identity, 3*(1), 11–23.
Policy Innovation Unit (2000) (www.cabinetoffice.gov.uk/innovation/2000/winning/active/foreward.htm)
Powell, J., & Biggs, S. (2000). Managing old age: The disciplinary web of power, surveillance and normalization. *Journal of Aging and Identity, 5*(1), 3–14.
Rowe, J., & Kahn, R. (1998). Successful aging. *The Gerontologist, 37*, 433–440.
Sawchuk, K. (1995). From gloom to boom; Age, identity and target marketing. In M. Featherstone & A. Wernick (Eds.), *Images of ageing* (pp. 173–187). London: Routledge.
Social Exclusion Unit website (1997) (www.idea.gov.uk)
Social trends. (1988). London: HMSO.
Strategem. (2000). *Bulletin 5*. Wolverhampton: Better Government for Older People.
Taylor, C. (1989). *Sources of the self*. Cambridge: CUP.
The NHS Plan. (2000). London: HMSO.
Tornstam, L. (1996). Geotranscendence: A theory about maturing into old age. *Journal of Aging and Identity, 1*(1), 37–50.
Townsend, P. (1981). The structured dependency of the elderly. *Ageing & Society, 1*(1), 5–28.
Townsend, P. (1986). Ageism and social policy. In C. Phillipson & A. Walker (Eds.), *Ageing and social policy* (pp. 15–44). London: Gower.
Walker, A. (1986). Pensions and the production of poverty in old age. In C. Phillipson & A. Walker (Eds.), *Ageing and social policy* (pp. 184–218). London: Gower.
Walker, A. (1995). *Half a century of promises*. London: Counsel and Care.
Walker, A. (1996). *The new generational contract*. London: UCL Press.

Chapter 7
Active Ageing: Developing a Quantitative Multidimensional Measure

Laurie Buys and Evonne Miller

Introduction

With estimates that two billion of the world's population will be 65 years or older by 2050 (WHO 2002), ensuring that older people 'age well' is an international priority. In response to this global phenomenon of population ageing, numerous countries have turned to international directives promoting active, healthy or successful ageing, best epitomized by the popular World Health Organization dictum, '*years have been added to life; now we must add life to years*' (Walker 2002). Contemporary theoretical frameworks help challenge the traditional image of ageing characterized by physical and mental decline, dependency and social welfare provision, signalling a paradigm shift from conceptualizing ageing as survival in the twentieth century to a twenty-first century focus of ensuring quality of life in later years (Gergen and Gergen 2001; Grundy and Bowling 1999; Kalache and Keller 1999).

Gerontological research and theory have developed over the last 50 years from a predominately biological and medical focus on the physical reality of ageing to a more holistic approach, encompassing a wide range of health, social, psychological and financial factors. Traditional ageing research was clearly categorized into the three key domains of biological, medical and social sciences (Evans and Bond 1997); for example, initial theories of ageing, such as the 'wear and tear' theory and cross-linking theory of ageing, focused exclusively on the biology of ageing (Wong 2001), while social theories of ageing such as disengagement theory, activity theory

L. Buys (✉)
School of Design, Faculty of Built Environment and Engineering, Queensland University of Technology, Brisbane, QLD, Australia
e-mail: l.buys@qut.edu.au

E. Miller
School of Design, Queensland University of Technology, Brisbane, QLD, Australia

G.M. Boulton-Lewis and M. Tam (eds.), *Active Ageing, Active Learning: Issues and Challenges*, Education in the Asia-Pacific Region: Issues, Concerns and Prospects 15, DOI 10.1007/978-94-007-2111-1_7, and continuity theory focused on the psychological changes experienced by the people as they age (Putnam 2002). Contemporary theoretical frameworks of ageing, however, attempt to integrate the biological, medical and social sciences, emphasizing that well-being in later life is not solely dependent on physical health, but is influenced by social participation, psychological well-being, lifestyle and activities, financial resources, home and neighbourhood characteristics.

Contemporary Theoretical Frameworks of 'Ageing Well'

As Table 7.1 illustrates, contemporary theoretical frameworks of ageing – such as active ageing, healthy ageing, productive ageing and successful ageing – typically offer a positive, multidimensional approach which emphasizes the importance of maintaining and fostering the physical and mental well-being of people as they age. The focus has shifted to identifying the universal predictors of 'ageing well' and developing a key set of measurable indicators, with contemporary theoretical frameworks of ageing offering broad direction on the types of relevant issues and factors to be included. But, as Table 7.1 illustrates, although the frameworks share basic similarities in terms of fostering aspects of physical, emotional, social and economic well-being, each defines the process and priorities of the ageing experience slightly differently and has its own unique focus, strengths and weaknesses.

Perhaps the most well-known framework is 'Successful Ageing', which was originally developed by Rowe and Kahn (1998) and is fundamentally underpinned by a strong medical model with personal health being viewed as the key goal and an individual's choice and behaviour determining their health as they age. However, it has been criticized for applying the term 'successful' to ageing and for focusing on the impact of individual choice and behaviour on the quality of the ageing experience, thus downplaying the importance of broader societal influences and differential

Table 7.1 The differing theoretical frameworks for 'ageing well'

Framework	Definition
Active ageing	'The process of optimizing opportunities for physical, social and mental well-being throughout the life course, in order to extend healthy life expectancy, productivity and quality of life in older age' (WHO 2002, p. 12)
Healthy ageing	'Ability to continue to function mentally, physically, socially and economically as the body slows down its processes' (Hansen-Kyle 2005, p. 46)
Productive ageing	'Any activity by an older individual that produces goods or services, or develops the capacity to produce them, whether they are to be paid for or not' (Bass et al. 1993, p. 6)
Successful ageing	'Low probability of disease and disease-related disability; high cognitive and physical functioning and active engagement with life' (Minkler and Fadem 2002, p. 229)

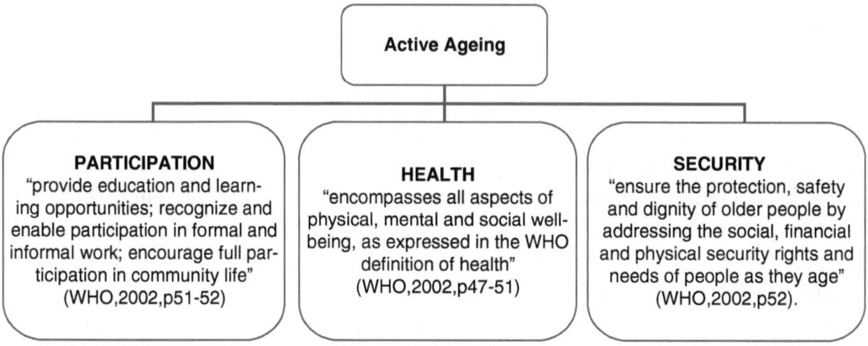

Fig. 7.1 The health, participation and security pillars of active ageing

access to resources (Holstein and Minkler 2003). Crowther and colleagues (2002) also recently argued that positive spirituality was a missing component to Rowe and Kahn's three-factor model of successful ageing. In both the successful and healthy ageing frameworks, physical health generally plays a predominant and central role. The productive ageing framework, however, reflects a move away from health and medical issues as the central focus. The concept of productive ageing was created to challenge the myth that productivity stops once a person becomes older, primarily focusing on the economic-based accomplishments and contributions of older people in terms of paid employment and volunteering (Bass et al. 1993). Critics of productive ageing, however, note that it excludes significant areas such as personal health and argue that the strict definition of productive activity means that some older people could be interpreted as 'non-productive and therefore, of lesser value' (O'Reilly and Caro 1994, p. 42). Overall, there is no one single definition of healthy ageing, which has been defined in a variety of ways with differing underlying assumptions, as it is multidimensional and covers a range of physical, cognitive and social factors (Hansen-Kyle 2005).

In order to overcome key criticisms of past frameworks and incorporate the key foci of successful and productive ageing, in 2002, the World Health Organization released its 'Active Ageing' framework. Figure 7.1 illustrates the three basic pillars of Active Ageing believed to be critical in encouraging people to remain active and independent as they age: health, participation and security. The WHO advocates a holistic perspective, arguing that multiple aspects of older adults' activities, specifically participation, health and security, intertwine to determine the quality of the ageing experience and that each pillar is essential in achieving and maintaining well-being in later life. Critically, the active ageing framework encompasses the health focus from successful ageing, the participation focus from the productive ageing, and through the security pillar, captures the importance of resources and the economic dimension for ageing well. The holistic perspective offered by the three pillars has positioned active ageing as the preeminent conceptual framework for investigating and understanding the impacts of multiple aspects of older adults' activities on quality of life and their general well-being as they age.

Challenges to Developing Measurable Indicators for 'Ageing Well'

Unfortunately, while each of these frameworks provides a valuable framework through which to conceptualize 'ageing well', they offer little specific guidance in terms of developing quantifiable indicators. First, this is due to significant debate over what to measure and what key factors constitute 'ageing well', with no widely accepted measure which enables a complete assessment of the key dimensions of 'ageing well'. Indeed, Tate et al. (2003) note there is '*no universally agreed-on standard or underlying theme for measuring success of ageing*' (p. 737), with Glass (2003) describing successful ageing as an immediately appealing, yet vaporous, concept. Second, as well as disagreeing over *what* to measure, researchers have traditionally tended to approach ageing issues from their own disciplinary background, that is *either* a medical, psychological, social, financial or cultural perspective to the extent that Bowling and Dieppe (2005) recently commented that '*the medical model is so dominant that few health professionals are aware of psychosocial ageing*' (p. 1550). While there is increasing awareness of ageing as a multidimensional experience, for practical reasons it is often conceptualized, especially by policy makers, in terms of singular health or social dimensions. Unfortunately, as Inui (2003) argues, the reality is that:

> The questions asked in such policy-making will not reside within one or another of the categorical determinants of health when, in reality, the choices contemplated are often tradeoffs among such radically different resources as bus passes, medications, city parks, senior citizens centers, and exercise programmes (p. 394).

The only way to make such policy decisions with limited resources, however, is to know which component should be prioritized. In order to advance the 'ageing well' agenda, therefore, there needs to be a methodology that provides a meaningful way of examining and measuring these conflicting ageing priorities. Without a clearly established quantifiable standard against which to evaluate or assess 'ageing well', however, there is limited consistency or comparability and no guidance for decision-makers.

The Australian Active Ageing (Triple A) Study: A Quantitative Multidimensional Measure[1]

The purpose of this research, therefore, was to develop a measure of the participation, health and security pillars of the WHO Active Ageing framework and to identify the factors which best support active ageing. The Active Ageing framework was selected as a guide as it seems to encompass most dimensions of ageing and has, to date,

[1] See Acknowledgements on page XXX.

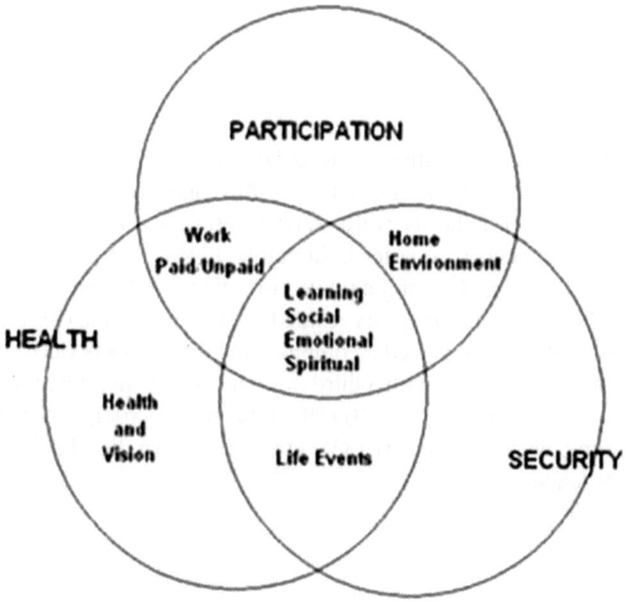

Fig. 7.2 The 'Triple A' domains of active ageing

avoided noticeable criticism. Notably, the WHO has provided little practical guidance regarding the definition or measurement of each pillar, instead, encourages nations to utilize the framework to identify and address the needs of their ageing population within the context of their own unique cultures and values. Thus, here we outline our experience of developing a quantitative multidimensional measure of ageing in Australia, the Australian Active Ageing (Triple A) Study.

Figure 7.2 illustrates the key domains of ageing explored in the Triple A Study, specifically the constructs hypothesized in the literature to define active ageing: work, learning, social participation, spirituality, emotional well-being, health and life events. It explores the multiple aspects that are thought to be significant to the experience of ageing in order to identify which variables contribute most significantly to quality of life for older people. Critically, as well as the more typical older study cohort, the Triple A Study deliberately captures the important 'baby boomer' group with participant age groups starting at 50 years of age. As the first multidisciplinary large-scale national study in Australia to explicitly explore 'Active Ageing', this is the first attempt to quantify the concept of active ageing, and we expect this framework and survey to prompt debate and be refined over time. This chapter outlines the methodology and measures developed to investigate and explore the domains of active ageing for Australians aged 50 years and older, with exploratory first and second-order factor analyses (which reduce the number of variables to uncover the structures and patterns of data) conducted to identify the domains most relevant to active ageing in the Australian context.

Method

Participants

A total of 2,620 older Australians – aged 50 years or older – participated. The average age was 62 years (ranging from 50 to 90 years), with women slightly over-represented (57%). The majority were married (66%) and living with a spouse or partner (66%), with nearly a quarter living alone (24%). Very few were separated (6%) or widowed (11%). Most of them lived in a metropolitan area (69%) and were born in Australia (76%). The majority resided in their own home (88%), had ceased full-time work (63%) and reported a combined income of A$49,000 or less (63%). Education levels were varied, with a third holding tertiary qualifications (31%) and nearly a fifth not completing Year 10 (19%). Overall, participants felt they were relatively healthy, with the majority (83%) perceiving that their health was 'good', 'very good' or 'excellent'.

Procedure

Participants for this national postal survey were recruited through the membership database of an Australian-wide senior's organization. In order to ensure a representative sample of older people in Australia, a stratified random sample of 6,000 address labels was generated from the organization's total membership pool to match Australia Bureau of Statistics population ratios in the six states and two territories of Australia. Participants remained anonymous to the organization. Approximately one third of the questionnaires were posted to individuals, with the remainder posted to a household where joint members were registered. When addressed to a married couple, the individual with the next birthday was instructed to complete the survey. To encourage survey completion, participants were offered entry into a prize draw for one of twenty $100 supermarket gift vouchers. A total of 2,655 questionnaires (44% response rate) were returned; after excluding incomplete surveys, analyses were conducted on 2,620 surveys.

Measures

The research methodology was quantitative, using a multidomain survey questionnaire. A 177-item survey covered the areas: paid and voluntary work (14 items), learning (33 items), social (11 items), spiritual (9 items), emotional (24 items), health (36 items), vision (6 items), home (11 items), life events (18 items) and demographics (15 items). A final open-ended question asked respondents to briefly describe what being actively engaged in life meant to them. The learning, social, emotional, health, vision, home and life event items were developed from existing surveys; in order to keep the survey to a manageable size, in most cases, an abbreviated version of full existing measure was utilized. The work, spiritual and demographic sections were developed by the research team. For brevity, the domains, questions and source of measures for the Triple A survey are illustrated in Table 7.2 below (a copy of the survey is available from the authors and example questions are also in the results section).

Results

Analysis

Statistical analyses were conducted using SPSS Version 14. To examine the factor structure of the constructs hypothesized to be associated with active ageing, exploratory factor analyses using the principal axis factoring method with orthogonal rotation were conducted on the seven key domains of Active Ageing: work, learning, social, spirituality, emotional well-being, health and life events. A first-order factor analysis reduced the original questionnaire items to a smaller set of independent factors, with a second-order factor analysis then conducted to explore how the domains formed higher-order constructs.[2] Only factors with eigenvalues (which measure the extent to which that factor explains the variance) greater than one were utilized. Cronbach's alpha coefficient factor (which measures the internal consistency/correlation between items and should be 0.7 or higher) was obtained, with similar loading patterns in the all-item second-order factor analysis. The results are presented by these domains (including an example of the type of questionnaire items in each domain) and then the results of the second-order factor analysis.

Domain Analyses

Paid and Voluntary Work

All items were correlated (KMO=0.74; Bartlett's test significant $p=0.000$), and five factors had eigenvalues greater than 1 (out of a total of 14). A three-factor solution (explaining 50% of the variance) generated the most comprehensible factor structure: *Engagement and Enjoyment in Paid Work* (explaining 21% of the variance and Cronbach's alpha coefficient of 0.88; items such as 'How many hours per week of paid work did you do in the last week?'); *Engagement and Enjoyment in Voluntary Work* (explaining 19% of the variance and Cronbach's alpha coefficient of 0.88; items such as 'How much do you enjoy doing voluntary work?' is 0.69) and *Engagement in Voluntary Visiting and Household Support* (explaining 10% of the variance and Cronbach's alpha coefficient of 0.53; items such as 'Do you do voluntary work where you do domestic tasks for someone in need?').

---

[2]For specific details on the factor analysis process, please contact the authors. Note that two rules were utilized in each analysis: Bartlett's test of sphericity and the Kaiser-Meyer-Olkin (KMO) measure of sampling adequacy.

Table 7.2 Domains, questions and measures for the Triple A survey

Domains	No. of questions	Measures
A. Paid and voluntary work	14	Fourteen questions developed by the research team asked about the degree to which participants were engaged in, and enjoyed, paid and voluntary work
B. Learning	33	Modified version of learning needs of older adults (Purdie and Boulton-Lewis 2001) asked participants their interest in learning new things (8 items), kinds of things they needed to learn (7 items), what they wanted to learn (7 items) and what kept them from learning (11 items)
C. Social	11	The abbreviated 11-item Duke Social Support Index (DSSI) (Koenig et al. 1993) was utilized to measure subjective support and social interactions
D. Spiritual	9	Developed by the research team, nine 5-point Likert scale questions measured spirituality, specifically spiritual beliefs and behaviours (belief in a higher being and regularly praying), spirituality in decision-making (reliance on intuition and personal ethics); and the importance of spirituality in life (searching for personal meaning, in control, contented with life, feel life is well spent, feel personal beliefs give meaning to life)
E. Emotional	24	Hoen et al.'s (1994) modification of Ryff's Psychological Well-Being 'How I feel about myself' 24-item survey measured emotional and psychological well-being. Participants were asked four questions from each of six categories: autonomy, environmental mastery, personal growth, positive relations with others, purpose of life and self-acceptance
F. Health	11 (36 items)	The SF-36v2™ (1992) Health Survey, a self-report generic health measurement, contains 36 questions to assess physical and mental health functioning. The SF-36v2™ measures eight dimensions of health, including physical functioning, role limitations – physical, bodily pain, general health, vitality, social functioning – emotional and mental health
G. Vision	3 (6 items)	Items from National Eye Institute Visual Function Questionnaire (Mangione et al. 1998). One common everyday task involving each of near and distance vision was selected, with degrees of difficulty reading the newspaper and driving determined
H. Home and Environment	11	Modified version of the maintaining seniors' independence through home adaptations: A self-assessment guide (Canada Mortgage and Housing Corporation 1993) assessed the home environment, with 11 of the original 24 questions on access, visibility, safety, usability, maintenance and comfort included
I. Life Events	9 (18 items)	Modified version of modification of recent life event and experiences questionnaire (Norbeck 1984; Sarason et al. 1978) assessed frequency and impact of nine events occurring over the last two years
J. Demographics	15	Fifteen questions, similar to those commonly used in surveys, were developed by the research team to collect information about socio-demographic variables

Learning

All items were correlated (KMO=0.84; Bartlett's test significant $p=0.000$), and eight factors had eigenvalues greater than one. Four factors were retained explaining 53% of the variance: *Obstacles to Learning* (explaining 22% of the variance and Cronbach's alpha coefficient of 0.88; items such 'Does self-confidence keep you from learning new things?'); *Independence and Security* (explaining 18% of the variance and Cronbach's alpha coefficient of 0.90; items such as 'Do you want to learn to discourage violence against yourself?'); *Openness to Learning New Activities* (explaining 8% of the variance and Cronbach's alpha coefficient of 0.90; items such as 'Do you want to learn to be open to new activities?') and *Interest in Learning and Current Events* (explaining 5% of the variance and Cronbach's alpha coefficient of 0.80; items such as 'Are you interested in environmental issues that affect Australia?').

Social

All items were correlated (KMO=0.90; Bartlett's test significant $p=0.000$). Two factors had eigenvalues greater than 1 and were retained, explaining 55% of the variance: *Satisfaction with Social Support* (explaining 41% of the variance and Cronbach's alpha coefficient of 0.87; items such as 'Do you feel you have a definite role in your family and among your friends?') and *Social Interaction* (explaining 14% of the variance and Cronbach's alpha coefficient of 0.67; items such as 'How many times during the past week did you spend some time with someone who does not live with you?').

Spiritual

The overall sampling adequacy (KMO) is 0.77, and Bartlett's test is significant ($p=0.000$). Three factors (explaining 70% of the variance) had eigenvalues greater than one and were retained: *Life Contentment and Control* (explaining 37% of the variance and Cronbach's alpha coefficient of 0.75; items such as 'Do you feel contented at this point in your life?'); *Personal Beliefs and Decision-Making* (explaining 21% of the variance and Cronbach's alpha coefficient of 0.66; items such as 'Do you feel that your personal beliefs give meaning to your life?') and *Spiritual Belief and Practice* (explaining 12% of the variance and Cronbach's alpha coefficient of 0.83; items such as 'Do you regularly meditate or pray?').

Emotional

The overall sampling adequacy (KMO) is 0.91, and Bartlett's test is significant ($p=0.000$). Five factors (out of a total of 24) had eigenvalues greater than one, with four factors (explaining 50% of the variance) retained: *Self-Belief* (explaining 29% of the variance and Cronbach's alpha coefficient of 0.80; items such as 'In general, do you feel confident and positive about yourself?'); *Life Coping* (explaining 8% of the variance and Cronbach's alpha coefficient of 0.77; items such as 'Do you often feel overwhelmed by your responsibilities?'); *Satisfaction with Relationships* (explaining 7% of the variance and Cronbach's alpha coefficient of 0.74; items such as 'Do you feel that you get a lot out of your friendships?') and *Personal Growth* (explaining 6% of the variance and Cronbach's alpha coefficient of 0.65; items such as 'Are you the kind of person who likes to give new things a try?').

Health

The overall sampling adequacy (KMO) is 0.96; Bartlett's test is significant ($p = 0.000$), and seven factors were retained (explaining 53% of the variance). An examination of item loadings suggests the following components: *General Health and Vitality* (items such as 'Is your health excellent?'); *Emotional Health* (items such as 'During the past 4 weeks have emotional problems prevented you from accomplishing all you would like?'); *Physical Functioning* (items such as 'Does your health limit you from walking one hundred metres?'); *Role Physical* (items such as 'During the past 4 weeks has your physical health limited the kind of work or other activities you do?'); *Mobility in the Home* (items such as 'Do you have difficulty in moving within some areas or rooms due to lack of ineffective handrails and grab bars in your home?'); *Safety in the Home* (items such as 'Do you have difficulty in keeping your home safe and secure from theft or intrusion?') and *Vision* (items such as 'Do you accomplish less than you would like because of your vision?'). The Cronbach's alpha coefficients were 0.89 for 'General Health and Vitality', 0.90 for 'Emotional Health', 0.90 for 'Physical Functioning', 0.94 for 'Role Physical', 0.59 for 'Home Mobility', 0.52 for 'Safety' and 0.46 for 'Vision'.

Life Events

The overall sampling adequacy (KMO) is 0.63, and Bartlett's test is significant ($p = 0.000$). Four factors had eigenvalues greater than 1 out of a total of 9. A two-factor solution (explaining 32.5% of the variance) generated the most comprehensible factor structure: *Experience of Challenging Events* (Cronbach's alpha coefficient of 0.46; items such as 'In the past year have you experienced a major unexpected financial hardship and if so how did it affect your life?') and *Productive Engagement in Life* (Cronbach's alpha coefficient of 0.29; items such as 'In the past year have you commenced any form of study and if so how did it affect your life?').

Second-Order Factor Analysis

A second-order factor analysis was carried out to explore how the 25 factors from the domain analyses formed higher-order constructs; eight factors with eigenvalues greater than 1 (orthogonal rotation) were retained, explaining 55% of the variance. Table 7.3 presents the factor loadings of the first-order factors on these eight factors (only first-order factors with loadings > 0.3 were included).

Table 7.3 Second-order factor analysis factor loadings

	Factor (2nd order)							
	1	2	3	4	5	6	7	8
Factor (1st order)	Social engagement and satisfaction	Activities and engagement	Self-belief	Life coping	Personal development	Emotional health	Experience of challenging events	Physical functioning and roles
Satisfaction with relationships (Emotional section)	**.849**	.266	.002	−.208	.019	.129	.023	.023
Satisfaction with social support (Social section)	**.653**	−.001	.182	.034	.105	.142	.069	.020
Life contentment and control (Spiritual section)	**.533**	.082	.339	.303	−.077	.247	.199	−.053
Obstacles to learning (Learning section)	**.426**	.051	.202	.386	.119	.109	.243	.292
Safety (Health section)	**.210**	−.056	.013	.096	.003	−.058	.168	.046
Vision (Health section)	**.147**	.036	.003	.055	.126	−.042	.120	−.006
Voluntary work (Work section)	−.027	**.715**	.113	.118	.158	.002	−.068	.074
Productive engagement in life (Life events section)	−.047	**.477**	.054	.159	.078	−.056	−.379	.165
Social interaction (Social section)	.219	**.444**	−.032	.036	.132	.068	.119	−.089
Spiritual belief and practice (Spiritual section)	.018	**.327**	.004	−.166	.012	.005	−.008	−.099
Visiting and household support (Work section)	.091	**.151**	−.004	−.106	.061	.024	−.037	−.085
Self-belief (Emotional section)	.167	.023	**.883**	−.059	.140	.105	−.033	−.068
General health and vitality (Health section)	.204	.061	**.219**	.135	.057	−.123	.168	.204
Life coping (Emotional section)	.304	−.063	.055	**.710**	.074	.175	.188	−.083

(continued)

Table 7.3 (continued)

Factor (1st order)	Factor (2nd order) 1 Social engagement and satisfaction	2 Activities and engagement	3 Self-belief	4 Life coping	5 Personal development	6 Emotional health	7 Experience of challenging events	8 Physical functioning and roles
Independence and security (Learning section)	.031	–.003	.028	**–.243**	.017	–.023	.012	–.014
Personal growth (Emotional section)	.039	.171	–.070	.106	**.675**	.004	–.089	.252
Interest in learning and current events (Learning section)	.082	.094	.239	–.029	**.517**	.007	–.114	–.037
Personal beliefs and decision-making (Spiritual section)	.278	0.179	.311	–.067	**.344**	.080	–.029	–.065
Openness to learning new activities (Learning section)	–.044	.082	.022	–.126	**.240**	–.007	–.026	.220
Emotional health(Health section)	.297	.083	.145	.294	.023	**.839**	.104	–.006
Experience of challenging events (Life events section)	.078	–.049	.051	.072	–.107	.169	**.634**	.036
Mobility in the home (Health section)	.080	–.007	–.040	.009	–.053	–.043	**.148**	.087
Paid work (Work section)	.056	–.113	.061	–.104	.074	–.035	–.057	**.520**
Physical functioning (Health section)	.013	.032	–.032	.116	.112	–.042	.030	**.341**
Role physical (Health section)	–.008	–.050	–.058	.018	–.049	.056	.088	**.328**
Percentage of variation 'explained'	**15**	**10**	**7**	**6**	**5**	**4**	**4**	**4**

The highest factor is in bold

The first factor, 'Social Engagement & Satisfaction', explained 15% of the variance and comprised of factors dealing with social and emotional elements of relationships and support. The second factor, 'Activities & Engagement', explaining 10% of the variance, comprised of factors dealing with engaging in voluntary activities. The third factor, 'Self-Belief', explaining 7% of the variance, comprised of items dealing with feelings of confidence and direction in life. 'Life Coping', explaining 6% of the variance, comprised of items dealing with perceptions of feeling overwhelmed by responsibilities and the demands of everyday life. 'Personal Development', explaining 5% of the variance, comprised of items referring to interests in 'learning new ways of doing things' and an engagement in learning and current events more generally. 'Emotional Health', explaining 4% of the variance, dealt with perceptions of emotional problems and depression. 'Experience of Challenging Events', explaining 4% of the variance, comprised of the experience of having to make major decisions regarding the future and financial hardships. The final factor, 'Physical Functioning', explained 4% of the variance and consisted of items regarding physical limitations such as the ability to walk certain distances, climbing stairs and doing household tasks. Social and life participation and mental/emotional health issues dominate the factor structure of active ageing, explaining 25% and 22% of the variance, respectively, with only a small proportion of the variance explained by physical health and security issues, 4% each.

Discussion

The overarching aim of the international Active Ageing framework is to inspire policy and programmes that appropriately address population ageing in countries across the globe. To our knowledge, this Australian Active Ageing (Triple A) Study is one of the first attempts to respond to this challenge and explicitly quantify the complex determinants of active ageing that enable engagement in life, investigating the extent to which health-related quality of life, social support, emotional well-being, spirituality, learning and life events. We defined, measured and predicted 'active ageing' in a sample of 2,688 older Australians aged 50–90, which provides an initial starting point for those wishing to quantify active ageing and understand the interaction of multiple aspects of older adults' lives that promote quality of life and well-being.

The findings resulted in eight distinct elements that appear to define 'active ageing', explaining 55% of the variance. Interestingly, social and life participation and mental/emotional health issues dominate the factor structure of this survey of active ageing, explaining 25% and 22% of the variance, respectively, with physical health (4%) and security issues (4%) explaining only a small proportion of the variance. With the majority of the variance in active ageing accounted for by issues related to social relationships, life engagement and mental/emotional health issues, our findings support an emerging body of research which advocates moving beyond physical health status when understanding and conceptualizing ageing and utilizing 'measures which focus on more than mental and physical health and functioning' (Bowling et al. 2002, p. 361). From a practical intervention point of view, the findings suggest that engaging older adults in personal development and engagement activities, which require neither good physical health nor significant financial resources, will foster the mental health element of active ageing and enhance the quality of later life.

The findings suggest that, for older Australians, the WHO's three key pillars of active ageing, health, participation and security, reasonably accurately capture their experience and expectations of being engaged with life. Notably, for many older adults, issues of physical, mental, social and financial health intertwine to determine their engagement in life and, hence, the quality of the ageing experience. The inter-connectedness of the participation, health and security pillars highlights the multifaceted reality of active ageing, emphasizing that while researchers have traditionally tended to approach ageing issues from either medical, psychological, social, financial or cultural perspectives, enhancing our understanding of the experience of ageing in the twenty-first century requires a trans-disciplinary and holistic approach. Indeed, there is an increasing awareness in the medical literature that ageing well is more than just good physical health, with Glass (2003) arguing that clinicians must:

> protect ourselves against the belief that successful ageing is impossible if disease and disability occur. If our concept of successful ageing includes dignity, autonomy, social engagement, and the absence of suffering, we will be better positioned to configure our systems of care to address the needs of older populations (p. 383, 2003).

With the literature on developing consistent and quantifiable indicators for active ageing in its infancy, this survey must be viewed as the first initial step towards conceptualizing, operationalizing and measuring active ageing. Further qualitative and quantitative research is needed to explore the validity of the active ageing framework and clarify the health, participation and security needs, expectations and experiences of older Australians and their counterparts in developing and developed countries. Notably, as participants were relatively 'young, healthy and wealthy' fee-paying members of a national senior's organization and not necessarily representative of the general Australian population as a whole, future research using representative and random samples is essential. While this first conceptualization of active ageing may require improvement and refinement over time, it is designed to encourage feedback, debate and discussion regarding what aspects of active ageing can and should be measured in different contexts. Our intention is that other researchers will also attempt to quantify active ageing in different international contexts, thereby facilitating understanding of the complexity of issues that intertwine, converge and enhance the ageing experience.

Acknowledgements The research was funded primarily by a QUT Strategic Collaborative Program Grant. Thanks to Nikki David (statistician) for help with statistical analyses and interpretation. The contributions of the Triple A team are also acknowledged: Lovie-Kitchin, J., Boulton-Lewis, G., Tedman-Jones, J., Nayak, R., Courtney, M., Edwards, H., Anderson, D. and Zlobicki, M.

References

Bass, S. A., Caro, F. G., & Chen, Y. (1993). *Achieving a productive aging society*. Westport: Greenwood Publishing Group.

Bowling, A., Banister, D., Sutton, S., Evans, O., & Windsor, J. (2002). A multidimensional model of the quality of life in older age. *Aging and Mental Health, 6*(4), 355–371.

Bowling, A., & Dieppe, P. (2005). What is successful ageing and who should define it? *British Medical Journal, 331*, 1548–1551.

Canada Mortgage and Housing Corporation. (1993). *A self-assessment guide: Maintaining seniors' independence through home adaptations*. Ottawa: Canada Morgage and Housing Corporation.

Crowther, M. R., Parker, M. W., Achenbaum, W. A., Larimore, W. L., & Koenig, H. G. (2002). Rowe and Kahn's model of successful aging revisited: Positive spirituality - the forgotten factor. *The Gerontologist, 42*(5), 613–620.

Evans, J. G., & Bond, J. (1997). The challenges of age research. *Age and Ageing, 26*, 43–46.

Gergen, M. M., & Gergen, K. J. (2001). Positive aging: New images for a new age. *Ageing International, 27*(1), 3–23.

Glass, T. A. (2003). Assessing the success of successful aging. *Annals of Internal Medicine, 139*(5), 382–383.

Grundy, E., & Bowling, A. (1999). Enhancing the quality of extended life years: Identification of the oldest old with a very good and very poor quality of life. *Aging & Mental Health, 3*(3), 199–212.

Hansen-Kyle, L. (2005). A concept analysis of healthy aging. *Nursing Forum, 40*(2), 45–57.

Hoen, B., Thelander, M., & Worsley, J. (1994). *Ryff's survey (condensed) "How I feel about myself"* (Report on the evaluation of effectiveness of a community program for aphasic adults). Stouffville: York-Durham Aphasia Centre.

Holstein, M. B., & Minkler, M. (2003). Self, society and the "new gerontology". *The Gerontologist, 43*(6), 787–796.

Inui, T. S. (2003). The need for an integrated biopsychosocial approach to research on successful aging. *Annals of Internal Medicine, 139*, 391–394.

Kalache, A., & Keller, I. (1999). The WHO perspective on active aging. *Promotion and Education, 6*(4), 20–24.

Koenig, H., Westlund, R., George, L., Hughes, D., Blazer, D., & Hybels, C. (1993). Abbreviating the Duke's Social Index for use in chronically ill elderly individuals. *Psychosomatics, 34*, 61–69.

Mangione, C. M., Lee, P. P., Pitts, J., Guitierrez, P., Berry, S., & Hays, R. D. (1998). Psychometric properties of the National Eye Institute Visual Function Questionnaire (NEI_VFQ). *Archives of Ophthalmology, 116*, 1496–1504.

Minkler, M., & Fadem, P. (2002). Successful aging: A disability perspective. *Journal of Disability Policy Studies, 12*(4), 229–235.

Norbeck, J. (1984). Modification of recent life event questionnaires for use with female respondents. *Research in Nursing and Health, 7*, 61–71.

O'Reilly, P., & Caro, F. G. (1994). Productive aging: An overview of the literature. *Journal of Aging Society Policy, 6*(3), 39–71.

Purdie, N., & Boulton-Lewis, G. (2001). The learning needs of older adults. *Educational Gerontology, 29*, 129–149.

Putnam, M. (2002). Linking aging theory and disability models: Increasing the potential to explore aging with physical impairment. *The Gerontologist, 42*(6), 799–806.

Rowe, J. W., & Kahn, R. L. (1998). Successful aging. *The Gerontologist, 37*(4), 433–440.

Sarason, I., Johnson, J., & Siegel, J. (1978). Assessing the impact of life changes: Development of the life experiences survey. *Journal of Consulting and Clinical Psychology, 46*, 932–946.

SF-36v2™. (2003). Health Survey ©1992: Health Assessment Lab, Medical Outcomes Trust and Quality Metric Incorporated All Rights Reserved. SF-36® is a registered trademark of the Medical Outcomes Trust, (IQOLA SF-36v2 Standard, English). (Australia) 7/03.

Tate, R. B., Lah, L., & Cuddy, T. E. (2003). Definition of successful aging by elderly Canadian males: The Manitoba follow-up study. *The Gerontologist, 43*(5), 735–744.
Walker, A. (2002). A strategy for active ageing. *International Social Security Review, 55*(1), 121–139.
Wong, T. P. (2001). An old question revisited: Current understanding of aging theories. *McGill Journal of Medicine, 6*, 41–47.
World Health Organisation. (2002). *Active ageing: A policy framework.* Retrieved April 18, 2005, from http://www.who.int/hpr/ageing/ActiveAgeingPolicyFrame.pdf

Part III
Provisions for Ageing in Parts of Asia and Hong Kong

Chapter 8
Chinese Ageism Lives On: Grassroots Reports on Elderly Learning in Shaanxi, Jiangxi, and Jiangsu

Roger Boshier

Discrimination Based on Age

After May 4th, 1919, Chinese peasant revolutionaries hitched their wagons to 'Mr. Science' and 'Mr. Democracy'. Today, Communist Party 'science' spawns huge engineering projects and a space programme. As for 'democracy', citizens are waiting. Is 'Mr. Democracy' the yet-to-appear 5th modernization?

Revolution was designed to overcome class-based oppression and feudalism. Yet, after 60 years of Communism, Chinese society still discriminates against people because of their age. Young Chinese women are urged to marry and have children (or risk being 'left on the shelf'). Employers are clear certain jobs are only for young people. Old people are too often seen as a hindrance to making money and get assigned menial or puerile tasks.

Ageism is the process of discriminating against people because of their age. In 'old' (pre-1949) China elderly people stood on a pedestal. In 'new' China, they are too often sidelined by modernization, knocked over in the money chase, and stigmatized. Much to the consternation of westerners, 50-year-old Chinese are regarded as 'seniors' and probably 'over the hill'. In contrast, the Canadian Charter of Rights forbids discrimination based on age. Hence, Canadian employers cannot advertise for 'a 25-year-old office receptionist'.

Among Chinese leaders and educators, there is a widely shared consensus that old people need hobbies, arts, or exercise to fill their day. Hence, local governments compete to ensure elderly citizens are docile, and the foreign friend will be taken to see the 'seniors university' or 'community centre' where older people hop, jump, cut paper, and sing. There is nothing wrong with hobbies and everyone needs exercise.

R. Boshier (✉)
University of British Columbia, Vancouver, Canada
e-mail: Roger.Boshier@ubc.ca

G.M. Boulton-Lewis and M. Tam (eds.), *Active Ageing, Active Learning: Issues and Challenges*, Education in the Asia-Pacific Region: Issues, Concerns and Prospects 15,
DOI 10.1007/978-94-007-2111-1_8,

But one of the worst things about being old in China is the way society constructs elderly people as a 'problem' and mostly irrelevant to modernization or making money.

Learning (or the lack of it) is at the heart of many problems impeding progress in the People's Republic. The task here is to shed light on learning among elderly people in China.

Purpose of This Study

Having regard to the foregoing, the purposes of this study were to:

- Analyse sociocultural impediments to elderly learning in China;
- Give voice to impoverished elderly persons in rural China;
- Argue the case for offering elderly learners serious intellectual work (not just hobbies and exercise programmes).

From Filial Piety to Irrelevance

In the Confucian state, older people were venerated and children expected to care for parents. Senior citizens were valued for their wisdom and experience. Traditional respect accorded to elderly people was dramatically eroded by the Communist proclivity for elderly persons to abuse power. As Long March veterans grew older, they used their advanced age to suppress rivals and build a gerontocracy. The current unwillingness to value elderly people partly stems from suffering triggered by political leaders clinging to power in old age.

Mao was born in 1893 and lost credibility after the death (by starvation) of 30 million people in the 1958–1960 Great Leap Forward. Knowing this, in 1965, the 72-year-old Chairman staged a publicity stunt to demonstrate his vigour and grasp on power. He entered the Yangtze at Wuhan and drifted (newspapers said 'swam') down the river. Lifesavers and photographers were stationed at strategic points. The Chairman's 'swim' caused a sensation, and soon thereafter, he launched the Cultural Revolution costing the lives of a further 30 million citizens.

Long March veteran Deng Xiao Ping was 85 years old at the time of the June 4th, 1989, massacre in Beijing streets. In May 1989, 'Deng Xiao Ping convened Party elders to take charge since the younger generation of leaders seemed unable to manage' (Nathan and Link 2001, p. 223).

On June 2nd, 1989, elders decided to use force to end the loss of face endured by having students camped in Tiananmen Square. On June 4th the world saw what happens when unelected, vulnerable, and poorly educated older men have an army of naive youngsters at their disposal. Yet, despite the trauma of Tiananmen, chain-smoking Deng remained influential until his death at age 93 years in February 1997.

Because so many citizens have been hurt by octogenarian leaders, it is easy to understand why so many twenty-first century Chinese people think older adults should be quiet. They should amuse themselves with hobbies and not cause trouble. But it is not so simple.

Unprecedented Numbers

The ageing process will be particularly pronounced over the next 40 years and impede the ability of China to surpass the USA as a global superpower. By 2050, China will have 330 million people aged 65 years or more – a number roughly equal to the current combined populations of Japan, France, Germany, and the UK. By 2050, the median age in China will be 45 years – much older than in other places.

There are roughly 100 million 65-year-old (or older) citizens in China today. There will be twice as many in 20, and three times this number 30 years from now. The ratio of working-age to retired people will shrink. In France it took more than 100 years to double the percentage of people aged 65 or more. In China, this is set to occur in only one generation – 'a pace and extent scarcely before witnessed in human history' (Haas 2008, p. 32). Who will care for this vast army of old people?

Chinese typically depend on filial solidarity to meet the needs of elderly people. Hence, leaders lecture citizens about family obligations. But, increasing divorce, the fragmentation of families (through migration), the money chase, and, in some cases, elder abuse have eroded filial piety and created instability. In addition, there is the '4-2-1' scenario where one child finds him or herself responsible for four grandparents, two parents and one child (seven people in all).

Disgruntled Seniors

Disgruntled elderly people threaten social harmony, and even old Communists resent the collapse of their consensus about how life should be lived. Hence, in October, 2008, Civil Affairs Minister Li Xueju urged all branches of government 'to learn about the difficulties and problems of (especially impoverished) seniors at a grassroots level and come up with effective solutions' (Official Vows to Improve Lives of Elderly Chinese, *Xinhua*, October 7, 2008).

Part of what alerted Beijing to disgruntled seniors were television pictures of 12,000 irate elderly people who lost relatives and homes in the Sichuan earthquake of May, 2008. Central government was also embarrassed by 79-year-old Wu Dianyuan and 77-year-old Wang Xiuying – forcefully evicted from their Beijing homes in 2001. They applied for a permit to demonstrate (on one of the authorized parks) during the Beijing Olympics. Along with 77 others, their protest applications were ignored. After applying five times, they were arrested and sentenced to 1-year of re-education through hard labour for 'disturbing the public order'. Mrs. Wang, 77 years old, is

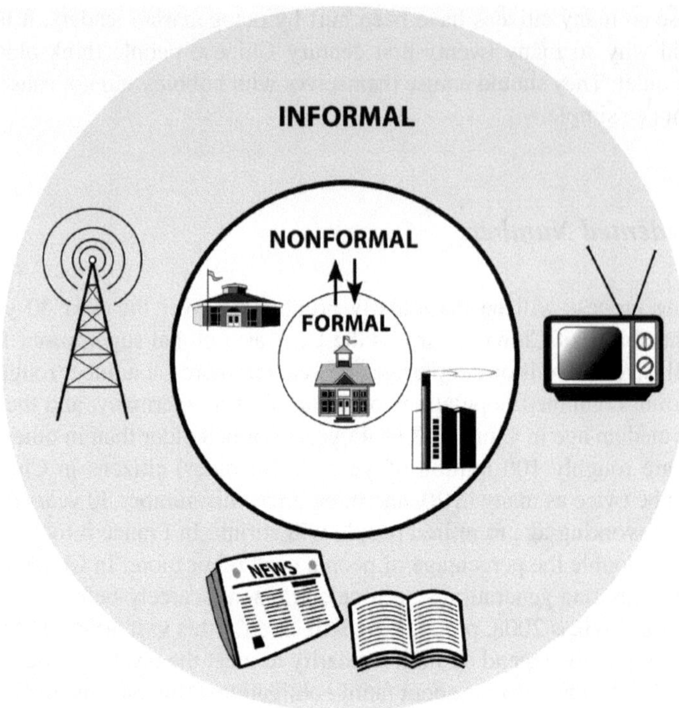

Fig. 8.1 Interrelationship of informal, nonformal, and formal settings for learning

blind and crippled. Once news of her punishment reached the Internet, authorities 'revised' the sentence. But it was too late. Beijing was hoist on its own petard.

Most elderly citizens in China live in poverty and without proper health care. Many are lonely, suicidal, or depressed. Like in most parts of rural China, in Wu Long village (Jiangxi) there are only very old and very young people. Grandparents are minding children while parents work in distant locations. The central government is aware of problems but stuck with depending on (often corrupt) local officials to implement policy

Money directed at the elderly has a bad habit of not reaching its destination. In January 2009 when the central government decided to invest four trillion yuan to stave off an economic downturn, a group of Party elders (led by Mao's secretary Li Ruihan) publicly worried about corruption. 'We are extremely worried that the privileged and corrupt will seize this opportunity to fatten themselves … and intensify social conflict', said elders in a letter to Beijing (Peh 2009, p. A2). Old cadres wanted checks and balances to dampen corruption.

Learning lies at the heart of nearly every problem in China. Resolving health-care, environmental, economic, land-use, corruption, and other crises requires learning – and lots of it. Not necessarily in schools and universities. Rather, as shown in Fig. 8.1, China needs broad-based, fluid, democratic, and participatory forms of learning in a broad array of informal and nonformal (as well as formal) settings.

Although Mao's revolution almost entirely depended on learning in informal and nonformal settings (see Boshier and Huang 2008, 2009b), in twenty-first century China, formal settings are the most prestigious and dominate educational discourse. Say the word 'learning' in China, and citizens typically equate it with formal education. Even adult education – which has a long and honourable history – is too often folded into authoritarian, top-down, and narrow strictures of Chinese higher education. Hence, Chinese typically speak of adult/higher education.

Too many elderly Chinese are illiterate and have only bleak (or no) memories of school. Only 6% of people in China aged over 25 years have a college education (Zhao 2009). The government has vast pools of money for dams and a space programme but not enough for elderly people.

Too many former employees of state-owned enterprises (SOEs) have had pensions looted by incompetence or criminal behaviour. Three-quarters of Chinese workers have no pension, and there is a massive shortfall in government obligations to the elderly. Even if the 2008–2011 global downturn is temporary, economic growth will not cover obligations to the elderly because China will turn old before becoming an advanced industrial state.

The government is under immense pressure and, in 2000, moved to cover certain pension liabilities left when state-owned enterprises imploded or were laid waste by corruption. Elderly Chinese need better health care, social support, respect, and money. Given the scope, severity, and incendiary nature of ageing in China, learning is a priority.

In 1999 when Beijing launched an initiative to build the biggest learning society in the world, officials were mostly thinking of China's ability to compete in the global economy (Boshier and Huang 2006b). Architects of the learning initiative were impressed by Senge's (1990) work on learning organizations. Launching a 'learning' (not an 'education') initiative indicates there is no chance of meeting China's needs through formal (particularly higher) education.

Lifelong Learning in China

Lifelong learning in China is a multifaceted and agile animal linked to ancient ideas but, as well, the cult of the new (Kingwell 2005). The Chinese interest in learning organizations, villages, towns, and cities stems from longstanding tendencies mixed with foreign influences.

In 1919 the May 4th movement assailed Chinese acquiescence to Japan and blamed Confucian culture for backwardness. Students from 13 Beijing colleges wanted a stronger western-style culture. 'They scoffed at the authoritarianism of the Chinese family, declared Chinese classical writing a hindrance to progress ... and embraced science and democracy as panaceas' (Terrill 2003, p. 103). The answer, they thought, was to reject Chinese tradition and look to the west. Education and learning were the focus. Hence, in 1919 university students went to Tiananmen and caused a ruckus.

Starting around 2000, authorities embraced lifelong learning. The first emphasis was on learning organizations (Senge 1990). In the next 2 years, it moved to learning communities. By 2004, there were vigorous efforts to build learning cities and a learning (Communist) party. By 2005, demands to build a learning society were supplemented by propaganda demanding a harmonious society. The need for harmony complements demands for learning (Boshier and Huang 2005, 2006a, b, 2007a, b, 2009b). Harmony is not possible without learning.

Few elderly people in China went to school, and despite official protestations to the contrary, there is still widespread illiteracy. Unlike city folk schooled in the delicate art of avoiding sensitive issues, peasants give their opinions about everything. They often present a 'very bleak picture of growing anger marked by sporadic protests and violent repression' (Becker 2008, p. 164).

Study Informants

Socio-economic status profoundly shapes the motivation and learning of elderly Chinese. With this in mind, Boshier et al. (2005) asked elderly Shanghai citizens in seniors universities why they were attending adult education classes. This survey, conducted with the *Education Participation Scale*, zoomed in on 'lost generation' learners using adult education to make up for schooling crushed by the Cultural Revolution. This was orthodox survey research involving multivariate statistics and many respondents.

For the present study, we interviewed four informants:

- Two relatively privileged people enjoying a good quality of life and
- Two impoverished (and illiterate) peasants from the countryside.

The task was to deepen understanding of what it means to be an elderly person in China by having them respond to questions about, for example, the happiest and saddest day of their life and how learning new things makes life harder or easier.

The first two informants had enjoyed distinguished careers in adult education. Now in their eighties, they both continue learning and assisting others.

Fang Jing

Mr. Fang Jing is the first of our well-off informants. Although born into a privileged family, he felt Communists were China's best hope and, from a young age, was an energetic educator. Although born in 'high-corner' Jian An district (in the Shanghai concession areas), as a child, he had no money or food. He is alive because of supplies given by a high school teacher.

Fang started learning calligraphy when he was 10 years old and is now a widely recognized expert. He graduated from high school in 1948 and immediately applied himself to the impending liberation of Shanghai. He first worked as an unpaid designer on an underground Communist newspaper aimed at youth. Nationalist police arrived and closed it. His first paid job was as an adult educator in night schools in liberated areas. At one time he was one of the youngest adult educators in China.

Fang became Director of Adult Education and then Principal of a spare-time school in Shanghai's Hongkou District. In 1979 he penned a letter about 'what's wrong' with Chinese adult education and mailed it to Party leaders in the Ministry of Education. The letter made suggestions about the rehabilitation of adult and vocational education and was later quoted in educational reform documents circulated throughout China. Fang Jing's plea for reform can be seen in his *History of Adult Education in Shanghai* (Fang 1999).

Fang is against rigid teacher-dominated forms of education. For him 'one size doesn't fit all'. His ancestors are from Songzhuang, Jiangsu Province, where he now counsels students and teaches calligraphy. At the back of his house is a fishpond and, across fields, men building boats for the Yangtze delta. Fang mentors young people seeking entry to university. His calligraphy studio is a gathering place, and on the wall outside, a granite stone lists Songzhuang young people sent to university with his assistance.

Fang has clear views about ageing and elderly learning. Along with manifesting the attributes of lifelong learning, he is a strong supporter of the arts and believes elderly people are capable of serious intellectual work and have a duty to support younger ones.

Madame Li Li

Li Li is our second well-off informant (Boshier and Huang 2009a). In 1926 Yin Xiusheng was born into a privileged Jiangsu family whose background was the antithesis of those sought by Communists. Her great-grandfather was a high-ranked inspector in the Qing imperial court, and her grandfather, a Chinese ambassador to France. She was born in Huai'an which had become an important prefecture when the Grand Canal was dug in 352 A.D.

In 1939 Japanese troops were pounding Huai'an. Japanese occupiers insisted citizens show respect by bowing. Mr. Yin refused to kowtow. Although only 34 years old and in good health, Mr. Yin was weakened by beatings and died. The indomitable Mrs. Yin was now a widow with six daughters.

Xiusheng was only 14 years old when her father died. With the encouragement of her elder sister, consent of her mother, and under the influence of Yin Chusheng, a cousin already working for revolution, she joined the Chinese Communist Party.

Knowing the mother was in danger, Yin girls tried concealing their identity by taking new names. Four of them were working for the New Fourth Army. The four most common family names in China are Zhao, Qian, Sun, and Li. Yin Xiusheng became Miss Li. Elder sister Yin Zhensheng changed to Sun Qun. Two others became Qian Yi and Zhao Heng. At the time, many people were using an alias to confuse enemies (Li 2005a).

Some of Li Li's most troubling experiences were in the 1941 Japanese mopping-up operation in Jiangsu (Li 2005a). 'I was assigned to work in northern Pincha. One day after breakfast, I was going out to work with a comrade named Tian Zhijiu. He was arrested by Japanese when walking along the dyke in Yangkou Village. By that afternoon his head was hanging in Pincha Town. A male university student was hiding in a cottage when discovered by Japanese troops. He refused to open the door so they set the house on fire and burned him to death' (Li 2005b, p. 169).

During the civil war, cadres like Li Li mobilized about three million people for the last big battle. Communists overwhelmed Shanghai on May 27th, 1949. General Chen Yi of the East China Field (formerly New Fourth) Army was informed he would be Mayor of Shanghai. In 1953 Li Li and her husband were invited to work for the Shanghai municipal government, then desperately short of competent cadres (leaders). On National Day (October 1st, 1953), they headed to Shanghai where she worked on Party discipline.

Li Li left the Party Discipline department in 1958 and spent 5 years as Secretary-General and Principal of Shibei High School. During the Cultural Revolution, she was paraded wearing a placard attesting to her lack of redness, denounced as a 'revisionist', and her name struck out with a large red cross. She was made to do the 'aeroplane' – lean forward with arms in an upright position for hour after hour. While in this painful position, high school Red Guards and Bureau of Education employees shouted insults (Li 2006a).

After the Cultural Revolution, she was tasked to revive adult education. Almost nothing remained after the Cultural Revolution. Infrastructure was damaged or missing; schools had been closed for 10 years; teachers were reluctant, missing, or lacking basic skills. The task was to 'build something from nothing' (Li 2006a). She also had to find pedagogies more effective and humane than memorizing banal quotations and yelling at people.

These days Li Li has no contact with official Shanghai. But having witnessed (and participated) in the best and worst aspects of Communist revolution, her views concerning the emancipatory possibilities of learning should be heard.

At age 84, Li Li is still a committed (though critical and questioning) Communist and patriotic Chinese. But ageism and suspicion of strong women severed her connections to those in power. Li Li is concerned by current trends. She worries about corruption and the single-minded pursuit of money, regrets the loss of the moral compass that once guided revolution, and thinks it difficult to build harmony without reconciling with the past (Li 2006b). After a life like this, she feels elderly learners deserve resources, respect, and meaningful roles in a rapidly changing society.

Granny Fu

After the Long March, Yan'an (in Shaanxi) was a hotbed of adult education. Because 99% of peasants and soldiers were illiterate, books were of little use. Hence, the Party used street theatre and other participatory methodologies. Yan'an authorities today turn on loud music at 7.30 a.m. and ballroom, fan, and sword, and other kinds of elderly dancers hop, skip, and twirl along the riverfront plaza. It is a continuation of a lively Yan'an tradition of staging outdoor theatre and educational events (see Boshier and Huang 2008, 2009b).

In 2008, Boshier and Huang (2009b) explored villages along the last miles of the Long March to find out how elderly people view life in the twenty-first century against the backdrop of Communist revolution.

Granny Fu was sunning herself on a stone seat outside her cave in Xi Tao village. She lives in a cave near Yan'an and is poor, illiterate, and charming. She is a skilled and loquacious cook. Grandchildren and great-grandchildren told neighbours foreigners had arrived, and as is so often the case in rural China, a crowd formed and an individual chat with grandma turned into group discussion.

On January 13th, 1937, a large group of Long Marchers arrived in Yan'an, and Mao set up housekeeping in a cave at Fenghuangshan (Phoenix Mountain) – in the 'old town'. Granny Fu remembers Red soldiers in her village. She and her sisters ran into caves and hid. Villagers could never tell whether soldiers were Nationalist, Communist, Japanese, or the militia of a warlord. Soldiers always meant trouble. Because Fu's father was a landowner, arrival of the Reds meant family land was confiscated. Fu's dad decided to cooperate and ended up with a high position in the Communist government.

Xi Tao is picturesque in a dry and dusty way. Most people live in caves. Small pigs snuffle when disturbed. Almost every dwelling has a rack for drying corn in intense Shaanxi sun. Corn sustains animals in winter. But with spring festival imminent, being a pig is hazardous.

Granny Fu has 18 grandchildren and great-grandchildren and knows how to coax crops from unstable and arid loess. After a lifetime of illiteracy, she chuckles when asked what she would like to learn. She places little importance on her uncredentialled knowledge. For her, learning out-of-school is illegitimate. Her sons gave her a T.V. so she could see the 2008 Beijing Olympics. Changing channels is confusing and reception not good. But grandchildren like it, so it will stay.

Granny Fu is 77 years old, has a deeply lined face and worn hands. Intense Shaanxi sun and wind accelerate the ageing process although she has fared better than her cousins.

The saddest day of her life? The Great Leap when people starved.

The happiest? The birth of her children.

The biggest problem in the village? "No money ….!" "Corruption." "No health-care."

How about learning something new? Err, um ! Ha, hah! I am illiterate and so are my sisters and cousins (several of whom have arrived to listen to Fu and see foreigners).

Has she heard of the Internet? Yes, but does not know what it can do.

Can she read "poison" labels on cans and bottles? No.

Health care? She has no insurance and cannot afford doctors. If necessary, she buys "medicine" up the street. It is not an issue. Her time will come, and when we (the foreigners) return, she may not be there.

"What needs to be done to improve life in the village?"

"Appoint an official from here," she says, evoking smiles and murmurs of approval from the crowd.

Wu Rongyu

Wu Long village is in a green valley below Lushan in eastern Jiangxi province. There are no roads, motor vehicles, or dust. Wu Rongyu lives in an adobe brick house with his mother. Visitors normally walk to the village along a river valley, but with the assistance of a local woman, we took a shortcut over a hill. The first person we found was Wu – sitting outside his house peeling husks from tea buds.

Wu said he was old and, when it came to learning, had few options. He was wearing a threadbare PLA jacket, had few remaining teeth, lived in extreme poverty, and, having failed in love, was now minding his old mother. Neither he nor Mrs. Wu had many clothes. Yet, they had found dignity in poverty and were happy to be photographed and talk about learning.

'Old' Mr. Wu was only 54 years old.

Thirty years earlier, a matchmaker from a neighbouring village had brought a girl. The father of the 'bride' wanted a five-table banquet for the wedding. Wu's parents could only afford a two-table banquet. Negotiations reached an impasse, and the girl's mother called off the wedding. The loss of face was too great.

'I will never marry', he said.

Wu's mother is in her 70s but looked more like 90.

Wu went to elementary school for 5 years and has two brothers and five sisters. The brothers have families and houses in the village. He does not leave the village because he is 'low skilled' and illiterate. He has an unidentified illness but makes a little money growing tea and vegetables – sold to an agent in the village.

The Wu house was built in the 1980s. It has bamboo rafters and curled (but broken) tiles on the roof. Many tiles have been blown onto the ground and broken. Sky is clearly visible through the roof. There is no heat other than the cooking stove and coal is unaffordable. Unlike Granny Fu's place in Shaanxi, there is no heated kang (bed) in Wu Long village.

Mrs. Wu cooks with wood. Firewood gathering is a major activity, and as local supplies get stripped, villagers go further. Water comes from a dank pond up a hill. There are several villagers suffering water-related illnesses. Lunch consists of steamed rice with a vegetable leaf on top. During our visit, they had little food in the house, and like so many others, Mrs. Wu remembered the 1958–1959 Great Leap famine as the 'worst days' of her life. There are rudimentary gravestones on the hill behind the house. Mrs. Wu's husband is out there somewhere.

Fifty-four-year-old Wu has heard about computers, movies, and books but knows little of the world outside the valley. He is a good candidate to learn something new. Yet, he considers himself 'over the hill' and 'not suitable'. Education is good for children but not important for adults. His views are constrained by mountains and poverty. Yet he is an attractive and affable man who chuckles at our questions and wonders why foreigners would find him interesting. As to the threadbare PLA jacket he wears, 'it is a long story'. This is the extent of his wardrobe.

After finishing with Wu, we visited other houses. In one there are two impoverished brothers struggling with goitre or mercury poisoning. Their job is to mind a water buffalo in the rice paddy. They are paid 1 yuan (about 18 cents) a day. Yet, children say they are not the poorest of the poor. A small boy takes us to the poorest man. Like a character from a Yu Hua novel, the poor man has a grumpy water buffalo as his only companion. The animal knows it is knock-off time and resents doing another circuit with a plough so foreigners can take photos. This man – the poorest of the poor – also claimed to be 'old' but was only in his 40s.

There were no nuclear families (mum, dad, and the one child) in this Jiangxi village. Instead, elderly people were minding children while parents worked in far-off cities.

Not far from Wu's place, loquacious and motivated youngsters were eager to condemn authoritarian teachers and cruelty in the local school. Taking advantage of foreigners willing to listen, they complained about being beaten and having their ears clipped by a science teacher. But, in the next sentence, they extolled the virtues of learning and education. When pressed to name their goals, boys wanted to join Yao Ming in the National Basketball Association and girls aspired to be pop stars in Beijing. Later, teenaged girls confessed they must be 'realistic' and study hard at school.

We Gave Our Youth to the Party

Millions of elderly Chinese feel abandoned by the state and enraged by the collapse of what was supposed to be Communist utopia. There have been numerous demonstrations by jobless workers and pensioners. In addition to demanding back wages, unpaid pensions, or health benefits, they are protesting the marginalization and abuse of old people.

In November 2000, railway traffic between Shanghai and Beijing was stopped by enraged elderly workers in Anhui. 'Some 3,000 retired workers from a factory in the northeast blocked the main entrance to the China Third Metallurgical Construction Corporation (Goldman 2005, p. 205). They held signs saying 'We Have Given Our Youth to the Chinese Communist Party'. 'We Have Been Abandoned in Old Age'. Other banners said 'We Have Asked For Help From Our Children But They Have Been Laid Off'.

Elderly citizens were not blaming the central leadership. Instead, they are protesting state-owned enterprises (SOEs) and corrupt local officials. Because of theft and corruption when disposing of SOEs, there is a legacy of anger, debt, and missing pension funds.

Rural-urban migration is not the answer to these problems. Yet, because disparities in wealth threaten social harmony, the central government triggered the biggest migration in human history. As a result, families are fragmented, and more often than not, elderly people were left in villages as childminders. Grandparenting is a respected tradition in China. But tensions develop between traditional-rural grandparents and children carrying MP3 players and other accoutrements of modernization. This situation is graphically portrayed in the extraordinary Canadian-Chinese film co-production entitled *Last Train Home.*

There is an 18-year-old waitress from Anhui in a favourite Shanghai restaurant. Her sister works in another place and her brother in a Fujian factory. Her father works in Hangzhou, but she does not know his job. Her mother and grandmother are back in the Anhui village struggling with a farm. If lucky she sees them during the Spring Festival. But, if, as has happened, weather makes travel impossible, she must wait another year. For her, 'family' is just a memory.

As a result of the global economic downturn, railway stations are jammed with unemployed farmers returning to villages. Back in the village, it is good for returnees to be reunited with their (often hurt and angry) children. But many yearn for the city and some are drawn to crime. Disgruntled returnees are (and are not) good candidates for learning. It will take patience and inspired leadership to turn the economic downtown into a chance to learn something new. Yet the need has never been greater.

Gaps dividing rural and urban China threaten social cohesion. The crowd at Granny Fu's place in Shaanxi or Wu's leaky house in Jiangxi claim poverty is their biggest problem. The United Nations Development Program (UNDP) thinks poor people in China might be getting poorer. Health costs are responsible for 33% of what UNDP calls the 'new poverty'.

Concerning elderly learning, it is better to encourage local initiatives rather than top-down formulaic programming from Beijing. In rural China there are more than a billion people like Granny Fu and Mr. Wu scattered through an area the size of the USA. News about their lives rarely reaches cities. There has to be a focus on learning in the countryside and respect for the elderly and their uncredentialled knowledge. Do answers to their problems reside in learning villages?

Shuang Yu Learning Village

There is no grand template for elderly learning in China. Instead, only a patchwork quilt of pilot projects. But, all over China, bemused officials are being told to foster learning. Many are highly motivated and genuinely committed. They mean well but most do not know what to do.

The author was the only foreigner at a conference for high Party officials held in revolutionary Jiangxi (Boshier 2004). Others included the Vice-President of the Central Party School (Sun 2004), mayors, municipal officials, and Beijing-based architects of the learning initiative. In a keynote address, Zhong (2004), Deputy Editor of *Study Times*, urged delegates to give up the notion that there is 'one right way' to foster learning in China. Even so, pragmatic Party leaders had one pressing question for the foreigner: 'How do we build a learning village?'

Shuang Yu is the answer. It is an imaginary village in central China committed to making learning the central focus of rural life. Village activists were convinced economic prosperity would not reach their village until there was a better sense of social solidarity in the community.

They thought it important for people to learn about computers, welding, small engine maintenance, Internet, health and safety, history, art, politics, and business, but also understand larger issues behind what they were doing. Their 'Learning Alliance' conducted two consultations with local people. By sitting in a circle and writing on large pieces of paper, they came up with this learning code. Later, it was made into a wall poster and erected in Renmin Park.

The learning code was like the constitution of the Shuang Yu learning village:

- Shuang Yu is committed to all forms of learning.
- Everyone should engage in learning.
- Those who missed school merit special consideration.
- Educated girls become educated women.
- Learning occurs everywhere (not just in schools).
- Citizens should help each other.
- The Communist Party is a learning partner.
- Learning for work is no more important than learning for life.
- Learning should be collaborative, not competitive.
- Learning should be fun.
- Exams are useful but not always necessary.
- Elderly people are a valuable resource, and special steps are needed to involve them.

These inland Chinese wanted their learning village to foster vertical and horizontal integration within the context of lifelong learning (Boshier 1998). The situation can be portrayed like this. Learning should occur from cradle to grave. This is the *lifelong* dimension of the learning village. But, as well, there should be a more harmonious relationship between formal educational settings (like schools) and nonformal (out-of-school) ones like the workplace, home, or community. In addition, there are informal settings for learning which, in HIV/AIDS and other kinds of campaigns, are sometimes the only available option. This is the *life-wide* dimension of the learning village.

Figure 8.2 maps settings for learning. Most emphasis is usually on the education of young people in formal settings – the school (lower right zone). In a learning village, there has to be a more equal distribution of resources and emphasis on each zone. Hence, there would be as much emphasis on the learning of young people in nonformal (the lower left zone) as in formal settings (lower right zone). As well, there would be a considerable emphasis on the learning of older people (adults) in formal (upper right zone) and nonformal settings (upper left zone).

Each quadrant is the same size as the other. In a learning village, there would be a more or less equal amount of emphasis on learning in each zone. Formal and nonformal settings for learning are shown as clouds because they often overlap. Determined efforts to foster learning (such as during the SARS or avian flu crises in China) involve simultaneous use of all settings.

Shuang Yu organizers felt social had to come before human capital. In other words, people would be better able to respond to rural life, the economic downturn, and pressures of market socialism if they felt good about themselves, had close friends, support networks, and were active learners. Instead of training people or inculcating skills, the task was to nurture social solidarity, physical, and psychological health.

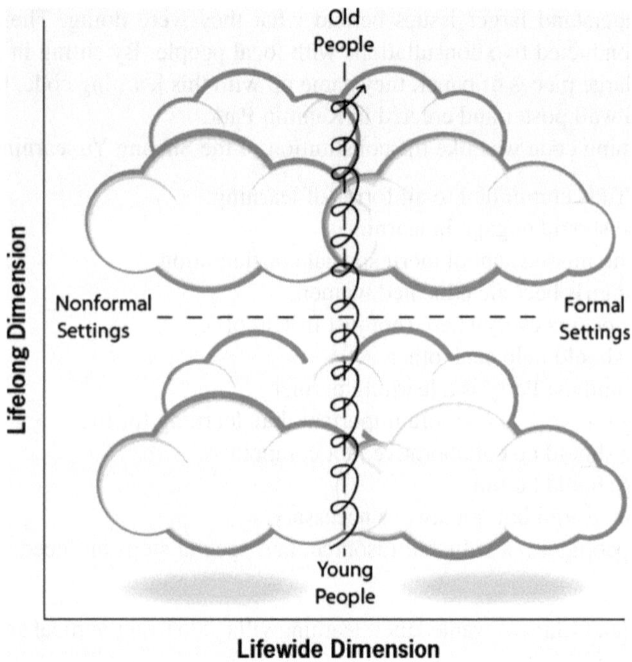

Fig. 8.2 Settings for lifelong learning

Architects of the learning village were determined to get young, middle-aged, and elderly people learning together. On the horizontal dimension, they defined learning broadly. Schools would be there but not take the lead. Throughout the first six meetings of the Alliance, Fig. 8.2 remained on the wall. Like Chairman Mao, Shuang Yu villagers were not enamoured with education in formal settings. All celebrated and had benefited from learning in informal or nonformal (out-of-school) settings.

The first task was to identify learners and teachers. They secured a map of the village, divided it into zones, and each member of the Alliance went 'door knocking'. Each person in the house – men, women, and children – was asked two questions. 'What would you like to learn?' 'What can you teach?' Many adults laughed at the idea they could teach anything and were surprised to hear villagers asking about their needs.

The contours of Shuang Yu were described in detail by Boshier and Huang (2007b). Here are some of the learning activities:

- Community reading programme
- Girls role model programme
- Old comrades learning project
- We learn, we teach
- Reading box scheme

- Village cinema
- Kites and flight
- Counselling centre
- Shuang Yu heritage museum
- Stop-smoking campaign
- Shuang Yu learning radio
- Shuang Yu diaspora support network (DSN)
- Shuang Yu 'bring-one, take-one' book exchange
- Homework-help project
- Shuang Yu pen pal project
- Olympic history wall poster project

A small but energetic group of Shuang Yu senior citizens felt the last years of life should involve significant learning. They used cards and pens to identify what they wanted to learn. Numerous elderly people wanted to learn how to use a computer. Several had grandchildren (even great-grandchildren) overseas or in other parts of China. Computers were the way to reach distant relatives. Some learners wanted to use the Internet for genealogy. As well as computers, seniors wanted to learn more about Chinese art and history.

Some were keen to do heritage conservation projects. For example, warehouses along the waterfront were more than 300 years old and mostly derelict. Could old comrades, assisted by younger members of the community, restore Shuang Yu's heritage for community purposes?

Some artefacts had been damaged by Red Guard vandalism. A few old comrades felt young people were alienated by modernization and the allure of cities. Using the Marxist maxim 'dig where you stand', they felt it important everyone know the genealogy of their community and family history. Hence, as well as riverfront warehouses, old comrades identified the following for action:

- Abandoned steam-powered farm machinery
- The old post office on Pearl St.
- The no-longer used People's Theatre
- Old shacks of unknown origins in the bush near Emperor's Rock
- A seventeenth century (and beautiful) little stone bridge over a creek near the big river
- The derelict house of Shuang Yu's most famous citizen, an eighteenth century writer, scholar, and artist

Shuang Yu is primarily a triumph of imagination. Yet organizers were stuck on the horns of numerous dilemmas. Should they share their experience with others? Should they allow a focus on social capital to be eroded by demands for workplace learning? Should they allow volunteer (and often elderly) 'teachers' to deliver 'give-'em-hell' non-participatory lectures? And what about scholars doing 'research' in the village? Should they risk becoming another Dazhai? (one of Mao's 'model communes' –a kind of Disneyland – from which others were supposed to learn). And what about the economic downturn? What did it mean?

As the third year ended, and Shuang Yu settled into a rugged winter, farmers lit smoke pots to protect fruit trees and members of the Learning Alliance scrubbed out premises on Xin Hua Street. Many people were pleased there was little resemblance between Shuang Yu learning village and teacher-centred, top-down, exam-oriented education as it plays out in Chinese schools or universities. In Shuang Yu the focus was on fluid and participatory forms of learning.

In the west, advocates of learning villages talk a lot about theory. But few put on boots and operationalize a complex idea like 'learning'. In Shuang Yu, villagers figured out practical ways to implement abstract ideas like 'lifelong education' or 'learning village'. Most important, elderly villagers have prominent roles. After years of being marginalized, several elderly people emerged as leaders. Among many notable triumphs is the Shuang Yu seniors choir.

Conclusions

Elderly learning in China is bound up with broader questions about human rights, filial piety, missing pension funds, and whether urban migration is the way to build a modern state.

After talking with informants and observing learning programmes involving Chinese seniors, the author reached these conclusions:

1. *The 'lost generation' created by the Cultural Revolution is a formidable challenge to those responsible for fostering elderly learning.*

   By 1966 Mao Zedong was convinced bourgeois culture had to be replaced by working-class values. Hence, the Cultural Revolution was launched in Shanghai on November 10th, 1965. Because faculty, curricula, and admission procedures were deemed traditional and bourgeois, university campuses were soon the scene of violence, strikes, murder, and suicide.

   The Cultural Revolution had an enormous impact on those who came of age in late 1960s. Urban high schools were closed, formal education suspended, and urban youth sent to the impoverished countryside. By 1977 when it ended, 20 million urban youth had lived a hard rural life for years. Millions of careers were postponed and lives ruined.

   Those damaged became a 'lost generation', and it is hard to find anyone in China willing to defend what happened. Public discussion concerning it is rare, and there is little research on why people did what they did. More than 20 million people were deprived of formal education and now want to make up lost ground through elderly learning. The Communist Party would rather forget the '10 years of catastrophe' and move on. But there is an enormous potential for fostering learning among citizens hurt by the Cultural Revolution.

   There is an enduring legacy of bitterness, disillusionment, and frustration. For advocates of elderly learning, it spawned an enormous cohort of potential participants. Today, the lost generation are involved in elderly learning and, because of their youthful experiences, need special forms of respect and expertise.

2. *Instead of being discursively constructed as 'dependants', older adults in China should be valued and respected. As active and informed citizens, they are vital to building a harmonious society.*

   Elderly people are capable of doing more than amusing themselves with hobbies. Having lived through political tumult, they understand what is needed in a harmonious society. There are millions of formally uneducated Chinese citizens (like Granny Fu) with considerable but uncredentialled knowledge of many things. There are also many educated people like Fang Jing and Li Li with attitudes and skills needed in times of rapid change. Although old people are repeatedly told learning is 'for kids', the appetite for new knowledge never disappears. Elderly people need warm, welcoming, respectful, and enjoyable learning spaces. Nobody wants to be a 'problem'.
3. *There are exemplary learning programmes for older adults but a habitual tendency to locate them within formal education.*

   Because of the historic importance and prestige attached to formal education in China, officials too often force learning activities into the framework of formal education. With teachers in charge, learners are silenced and trapped behind desks. Very few Chinese educators understand participatory learning, and most teachers dare not risk using group work, games, discussion, role playing, and other participatory processes. Because old people have a vast repository of experience, it is important to use it. It will be a challenge for Chinese to give up historic notions of 'teaching' and, in their place, develop a culture of 'learning'. Even in Hong Kong, the biggest elderly learning initiative focuses on creating university classroom spaces where there are few attempts to abandon traditional commitments to lecturing in favour of fostering learning in a manner better attuned to the needs and predilections of older adults.
4. *Too many Chinese officials have prejudicial ideas about elderly persons. Instead of fostering docility, officials should stress active citizenship.*

   The author has visited centres where elderly people are chopping paper, painting, making music, doing tai chi, and other forms of exercise. In some places, experienced, thoughtful, and intelligent people have been reduced to making paper birds. Hobbies, arts, and exercise are all good. But there are additional options. In Shanghai, retired adult educators who formed the Ming De Learning Organization Research Institute write reports, do serious intellectual, and help municipal governments embrace a culture of learning. Among their clients are Jiu Jiang City and the historic Lushan resort – the 'learning mountain' in eastern Jiangxi (Boshier and Huang 2006a). Elderly people dominate computer facilities at Shang Cheng Community College (Hangzhou) where they are writing local and family histories, researching science projects, exchanging documents with family members living abroad, cooking up heritage conservation projects, planning sports events, creating business plans, studying film, participating in online chat, consulting foreign newspapers, and writing biographies, autobiographies, and novels. Hobbies are good. But many elderly people need and enjoy intellectually challenging activities and projects. Old revolutionaries are not overly fascinated by paper birds!

5. *There are innovative elements in the national learning initiative. But little is available to senior citizens in rural areas. Solutions reside in communities.*

   Solutions to what ails elderly people in China lie inside communities. In most places there are motivated people like Li Li and Fang Jing – capable and ready to provide literacy and other kinds of assistance to people like Mr. Wu and Granny Fu. Small-scale projects adapted to local circumstances work better than grand plans implemented from above. There also have to be concerted efforts made to have isolated villages learn from each other. Along with others, Fujian activists associated with the journal *Lifelong Education* (published by the Fujian Association of Lifelong Education for All) are doing a good job publicizing examples of innovative learning perspectives and projects. Because Chinese adult has always been regarded as a subset of higher education, there is also a need to keep the focus on people learning together. Instead of dwelling on policy announcements and leadership theatrics, activists and researchers need to dwell in the grassroots.

6. *People involved with fostering elderly learning in China need arenas wherein they can gather and exchange ideas.*

   Places like Shuang Yu or the Shang Cheng Community College in Hangzhou have valuable experience worth sharing. Organizers of events called to share experience should be certain their processes exemplify optimal principles of learning. In too many Chinese conferences, the audience sits in silence or doze while high officials and 'leaders' read from text or stumble through a Powerpoint snoozefest. The sharing process should be enlivening – not deadening. It is not acceptable to give lectures about the need for participation.

References

Becker, J. (2008). *Dragon rising: An inside look at China today*. New York: National Geographic.

Boshier, R. W. (1998). The Faure report: Down but not out. In P. S. Jarvis, J. Holford, & C. Griffin (Eds.), *Lifelong learning in the learning society* (pp. 3–20). London: Kogan Page.

Boshier, R. W. (2004, November 20–21). *Black cat, white cat? Mice are nice. But learning matters more*. Proceedings of the Municipal Government National Conference Jiu Jiang on Learning Cities, pp. 28.

Boshier, R. W., & Huang, Y. (2005). The Shanghai-seven: Reflections 21 years after the ICAE meeting in Shanghai. *Convergence, 38*(2), 5–27.

Boshier, R. W., & Huang, Y. (2006a). Building for the future by expatiating the past: High drama from the summit of China's learning mountain. *International Journal of Lifelong Education, 25*(5/6), 351–367.

Boshier, R. W., & Huang, Y. (2006b). Is the Chinese learning initiative the long-awaited 5th modernisation? *Planning and Changing: An Educational Policy and Leadership Journal, 37*(1 & 2), 56–70.

Boshier, R. W., & Huang, Y. (2007a). Untold story of foreign devil adult educators in Shanghai silk factories, 1920 to 1949. *Adult Education Quarterly, 57*(4), 329–345.

Boshier, R. W., & Huang, Y. (2007b). Vertical and horizontal dimensions of China's Shuang Yu learning village. *Studies in Continuing Education, 29*(1), 51–70.

Boshier, R. W., & Huang, Y. (2008). Hey there Edgar Snow, what happened to the *Red Star* over Yan'an? *Convergence, 41*(4), 79–102.

Boshier, R. W., & Huang, Y. (2009a). Li Li: Communist revolutionary, adult educator, lifelong learner. *Studies in Continuing Education, 31*(1), 45–59.

Boshier, R. W., & Huang, Y. (2009b). More important than guns: Chinese adult education after the long march (1936–1939). *Adult Education Quarterly, 60*(3), 1–19.

Boshier, R. W., Huang, Y., Song, Q., & Song, L. (2005). Market socialism meets the lost generation: Motivational orientations of adult learners in Shanghai? *Adult Education Quarterly, 56*(3), 201–222.

Fang, J. (1999). *History of adult education in Shanghai*. Hong Kong: Wahha Culture Publisher.

Goldman, M. (2005). *From comrade to citizen: The struggle for political rights in China*. Cambridge: Harvard University Press.

Haas, M. L. (2008, August). Pax Americana Geriatrica. *Miller-McCune Magazine*, pp. 30–39

Kingwell, M. (2005). The city of tomorrow: Searching for the future of architecture in Shanghai. *Harpers Magazine, 310*(1857), 60–71.

Li, L. (2005a, June 14). Telephone interview by Yan Huang.

Li, L. (2005b). A girl in the new 4th army. In *Department of Old Party Cadres. War flame years: Collection of memoirs and articles by retired Party cadres of Shanghai Departments of Sciences and Education in celebration of the 60th anniversary of victory in the anti-Japanese War* (pp. 168–170). Shanghai: Department of Science and Education.

Li, L. (2006a, October 19). Face-to face interview by Roger Boshier, Yan Huang and Julian Boshier, Shanghai Education Hotel.

Li, L. (2006b, December 10). Telephone interview by Yan Huang.

Nathan, A. J., & Link, P. (Eds.). (2001). *The Tiananmen papers compiled by 'Zhang Liang'*. London: Little Brown.

Peh, S. H. (2009, March 14). Stimulus, but for whom? *The Straits Times*, p. A2.

Senge, P. (1990). *The fifth discipline*. New York: Doubleday.

Sun, X. X. (2004, November 20–21). *How the party school views the learning city*. Proceedings of the Municipal government National Conference Jiu Jiang on Learning Cities, pp. 51–59.

Terrill, R. (2003). *The new Chinese empire: And what it means for the United States*. New York: Basic Books.

Zhao, Q. H. (2009, February 28). *Public engagement key to better image* (Report of a speech by the Spokesman of the National Committee of the Chinese People's Political Consultative Conference). *China Daily, 29*(8998), p. 1.

Zhong, G. X. (2004, November 20–21). *Building the learning city*. Proceedings of the Municipal government National Conference Jiu Jiang on Learning Cities, pp. 51–59.

Chapter 9
Elderly Learning in Chinese Communities: China, Hong Kong, Taiwan and Singapore

Ernest Chui

Introduction

While the world has recently witnessed the ascendancy of China as a looming large economy, it should also be noted that Chinese culture, in its various manifestations, has also been embraced around the world. There has been increasing receptivity to Chinese herbal medicine, acupuncture, Tai Chi and martial art, calligraphy and not least the Chinese official language of Putonghua. The emergence of the Confucius Academy in various countries has also revealed the increased popularity and revival of traditional Chinese Confucian cultural values and practices. This is also couched upon the increased volume of Chinese migrants to various countries that makes the increasing presence and visibility of the Chinese community apparent to the host countries. On the other hand, as a general trend of the ageing population in many economically advanced countries, older people constitute an increasingly significant proportion in many Chinese societies. How best to meet with the challenges and opportunities presented by an ageing population has also been raised as an urgent agendum in many Chinese communities. One of the upcoming challenges would be the best utilization of the older population as a social resource instead of taking it as a problem or burden. In this connection, the promotion of 'active ageing' would be a possible solution. Research around the world has confirmed the merit and function of continued learning in promoting active ageing (Glendenning 2001; Boulton-Lewis et al. 2006; Withnall 2006). In this regard, elder learning could be one of the areas that deserves serious investigation. In this chapter, elder learning in four Chinese countries/regions – China, Taiwan, Hong Kong and Singapore – will be discussed. Here it should be clarified that as ethnic Chinese constitutes some 74% of the

E. Chui (✉)
The University of Hong Kong, Pokfulam, Hong Kong
e-mail: ernest@hku.hk

G.M. Boulton-Lewis and M. Tam (eds.), *Active Ageing, Active Learning: Issues and Challenges*, Education in the Asia-Pacific Region: Issues, Concerns and Prospects 15,
DOI 10.1007/978-94-007-2111-1_9, © Springer Science+Business Media B.V. 2012

Singaporean population (Singapore Department of Statistics 2010), Singapore would be taken as a Chinese community in this chapter.

General Background of the Four Countries/Regions

In the four countries/regions being considered, there is a difference in the extent of the ageing population. While Hong Kong ranks top in having 13% of its population aged 65 and above, Taiwan is the second (10%), Singapore is 9%, and China 8% (Population Reference Bureau 2009). With specific reference to the Chinese elderly population in Singapore, at end of June 2009, Chinese people aged 65 and above numbered 275,000, which constituted 9.9% of Singapore's Chinese population (Singapore Department of Statistics 2010).

With a Chinese cultural lineage, in the four countries/regions under investigation, three of them have adopted a paternalistic stance in promulgating legislations and policies that embody traditional normative principles that promote respect and care for the elderly. In China, Taiwan and Singapore, there are legislations on mandating children to support their parents (Chui 2007). For instance, in China, Article 183 in the Criminal Law (1979) and the Law on Protection of the Rights and Interests of the Elder (1996), with its Sect. II on 'Maintenance and Support by Families', are all relevant legislations stipulating the responsibility of adult children to support their parents and parents-in-law. In Taiwan, the government enacted the Senior Citizens' Welfare Act in 1980, which was subsequently revised and improved in 1996 and 2000. The Taiwan government has incrementally improved its provision of and/or regulation on elderly services in such aspects as medical services, subsidy to low-income elders, day care centres, home care services, and the like. The law, in addition to the Civil Law, stipulates the children's maintenance duty of their elderly parents and lays down penal codes to prevent elderly desertion and abuse. In Singapore, the Maintenance of Parents Act was enacted in 1995 with similar policy intent.

Apart from statutory provisions, governments in these countries/regions have also paid for efforts in promoting a generalized respect for the elderly in society. For instance, in China, the Chinese National Committee on Ageing, which was set up in 1999, is the central body overseeing older people's welfare. The Taiwan government reconstituted the organizational structure of the Social Service Bureau of the Ministry of Interior in 2007 to set up the Working Group on the Promotion of Elderly Welfare to oversee the coordination of the various government bodies (Taiwan Ministry of Interior, Social Service Bureau 2010). The Singaporean government has set up an Inter-Ministerial Committee on Ageing Population in 1999 to coordinate and oversee policies related to the older population. It also promulgates the Eldercare Master Plan (Singapore Ministry of Community Development and Sports 2001). Furthermore, a Committee on Ageing Issues was set up in 2004 to prepare for an ageing population (Committee on Ageing Issues, Singapore Government 2006). In Hong Kong, upon reunification with China in 1997, the inaugural Special Administrative Region government set up the Elderly Commission to demonstrate its emphasis on traditional Chinese virtue of respecting the elderly people.

Nonetheless, social development in these four countries/regions had been affected by their respective historical context, and that also had implications on their development of elder learning. Due to historical reasons, these four Chinese communities had been subject to similar historical trajectories of the prevalence of social upheavals, either due to natural disasters or wars that interrupted social development. The provision of education was met with challenges of insufficient infrastructure in terms of school premises, teachers and even basic teaching materials. This is particularly evident in China where the Communist regime was established only in 1949 after a prolonged period of civil war and Japanese invasion. In its early years, the Communist regime had met with natural calamities, like the great famine (1958–1962), coupled with political movements in the late 1950s to 1970s (e.g. the Cultural Revolution 1967–1976), which had incurred serious interruptions to the normal implementation of social construction, including education. Situations in the rural areas and the inland provinces would be even worse, given the relatively disadvantaged resource endowment in the underdeveloped regions. Taiwan ended its 50-year-long Japanese colonial occupation upon the close of the Second World War in 1945. The Taiwan government under the Nationalist Party, which fled from the Mainland upon the defeat by the Communist in the civil war in 1949, paid heed to economic reconstruction and buttressing the regime. Singapore got independence only in 1963 and had also been putting emphasis on economic development. Hong Kong, also suffering from war destruction and Japanese occupation before the War ended in 1945, had to concentrate on post-war reconstruction, especially in face of the large influx of refugees from across the Chinese border. Thus, compulsory, free primary education was only introduced as late as 1971.

Thus, in all these four countries/regions, social and economic reconstruction could only be revitalized after these upheavals were resolved. In the first few decades of reconstruction, economic development inevitably came to be the top priority of the ruling regime. In the social policy domain, education, which was taken as contributing to economic development by replenishing human resources, was also emphasized. Thus, Taiwan, Singapore and Hong Kong, which are also known as the 'Tigers' that had spectacular economic development since the 1960s, had been named as 'productivist' (Holliday 2000) or 'developmental' states (Tang 2000; Ramesh 2004) in which social welfare had been taken as merely supplementary and education was only regarded as contributory to economic development. This is evident in the heavy investment in education over the years in these countries/regions. For instance, in Singapore, as in 2009, expenditure on education constituted 24.8% of the total government expenditure, which was the highest single item (Singapore Department of Statistics 2010). As for Taiwan, education expenditure in 2009 constituted 12% of the total government expenditure – only second to defence expenditure (Directorate-General of Budget, Taiwan 2010). In Hong Kong, the figure reached 15.8% (in 2009), which is only second to 'welfare' (which included cash benefit on social security as Hong Kong had no social protection scheme until the setting up of a contributory retirement scheme in 2000) (Hong Kong SAR Government 2010).

As for China, since its economic liberalization only commenced in the late 1970s and the education infrastructure had been considerably disrupted in the social upheavals during the frequent political movements, especially the Cultural Revolution in 1967–1976, the Chinese government's investment in education is yet to pick up its momentum. Furthermore, as China is such a huge country that has to attend to multifarious concerns, education expenditure only constitutes 4.5% of the budget (in 2009) (Ministry of Finance, People's Republic of China 2010). In particular, given China's huge population pressure, government policies have focused on controlling population growth rather than on coping with population ageing (Poston and Duan 2000).

All these instances serve to sustain the postulate here that governments of all these Chinese communities could not afford to put much effort and resources onto catering for the need of elderly people, though there has been increasing awareness recently of the upcoming challenges of an ageing population. It should also be recognized that during those early post-war years, the ageing population was a 'non-problem' for these developing states, and thus, elderly welfare was certainly shovelled off the agenda. Albeit their possible divergence, these four countries/regions exhibit a commonality with respect to elderly education; that is, even though the government may deploy huge resources on education, emphasis had been placed only on providing education to young people, rather than adults, not to mention elderly people. This merely serves to substantiate the assertion here that lifelong learning for elderly people has been a late starter in social policy in all the four countries/regions under investigation here.

Although education policies and resources have not been particularly directed towards promoting elder learning, nonetheless, there are cultural roots that are favourable to fostering elder learning in these Chinese communities. In the first instance, the traditional Chinese cultural norm of filial piety is not confined to respecting the older members within the family but is extended to caring for the older people in society at large. Giving adequate provisions to older people is highly regarded as an individual as well as societal responsibility. On the other hand, Chinese communities largely have a Confucian cultural heritage. Confucius, China's most respected educationist, paid high emphasis to learning and regarded it as indispensable for becoming a virtuous person (Kim and Merriam 2004:117). Thus, learning has its intrinsic value per se instead of merely serving some instrumental functions of, say, occupational pursuits. In society, there is high regard for knowledge or intellectual achievements in the Chinese cultural normative order. This can be reflected by the prestigious positions enjoyed by the scholars or the 'knowledgeable' or 'gentry' class in the various dynasties in China's history. Educated people are, on the one hand, highly respected by the people and are expected to take up moral obligation to serve the community on the other. In contemporary context, educational attainment is certainly an indispensable personal asset for upward social mobility, as omnipresent in a meritocratic society. Thus, it is prevalent in Asian countries which have a Confucian-heritage culture (CHC) background that people generally display a positive attitude towards education, are achievement-oriented and are willing to spend a lot of their free time on studies (Lee 1996:25). Hence, it is logical to postulate that there is high expectation that people should pursue lifelong learning, as is practically feasible, to accomplish personal fulfilment. This is very much congruent with the western notion of lifelong learning that we are familiar with nowadays. Actually, there is a traditional Chinese saying that says, 'as you grow older, you have to learn as you age', which vividly spells the normative framework of Chinese people in maintaining a learning aptitude.

Motivation for and Mode of Elder Learning

Making reference to the tenets of industrial sociology and organizational analysis in understanding job satisfaction, we may conceive the underlying motive of elderly people (or people in general) in undertaking lifelong learning. Broadly speaking, we could identify 'intrinsic' and 'extrinsic' motives. Leung et al. (2006) identified 'expressive' and 'achievement' motivations underlying the 'intrinsic' motive and 'social' and 'instrumental' motivations underlying the 'extrinsic' one. The 'expressive' motive is based upon the elder learners' interest for sake of learning itself and their derivation of satisfaction directly from the understanding and/or acquisition of knowledge and skills. The 'achievement' motive is manifested as the learners' desire to succeed, for instance, in achieving a particular life goal of attainment. 'Social' motivation relates to the learners' wish to gain social acceptance or affiliation. Finally, 'instrumental' motivation designates the learners' motive to gain tangible reward or avoid negative consequences. Nonetheless, these four sub-types of the two broad categories are not entirely discrete. For instance, when an elderly learner engages in pursuing a learning programme that leads to a specific qualification, we could say that there could be multiple motives behind this: gaining friends when studying together, acquiring knowledge, proving his/her own competence, trying to be virtuous as a learner, getting a particular recognition to compensate for the loss during young or just learning for its own sake.

As aforementioned, there are specific socio-economic, political and historical trajectories that are peculiar to the four countries/regions under investigation that might have implications for the motivation for learning of the elderly participants in the countries/regions concerned. In the first instance, there is the incidence of the historical legacy of traditional Chinese patriarchal cultural norms and practices whereby women were disadvantaged, as compared to the male family members, in accessing formal education. For instance, in Hong Kong, not until 1971 was free compulsory primary education introduced, thus providing equal opportunities and access to formal education to both genders. Before that, sons could usually have better chance of attending schools at the expense of daughters, especially in poor families. China, being a socialist regime, has put emphasis on gender equality. However, given the relatively lower priority given to mass education as compared to economic development, there may still be the existence of relative disadvantage suffered by women in educational opportunities, especially in large rural areas, where the traditional patriarchal norms were more prevalent. On the other hand, as economic development had been considered as more important than social development, many people had been denied access to formal education when they were young. Thus, there could be the incidence of a 'compensatory' motive underlying many of the elder learners, especially the older women, when pursuing lifelong learning.

In terms of the mode or nature of lifelong learning for elderly people, there could be the conventional differentiation between formal, informal and non-formal modes. For the 'formal' mode, where qualification recognition, accreditation, entrance eligibility, credit transfer or advance standing, specific progression routes and the like are formally administered, they usually carry occupational implications. All these would make such a learning mode more restrictive. As for the informal and non-formal modes, such formalities could usually be waived, as people engaging in such learning would normally be concerned about personal interest and development rather than instrumental or pragmatic considerations. Such modes would allow more flexibility of entry channels and would therefore be characterized by a diversity of student population with a variety of learning styles and strategies. As in the four countries/regions, since many of the elderly people were deprived of formal education opportunities when they were young, there has been a considerable extent of low education level, or worse still, illiteracy, among the older population. Thus, there is a trend that elder learning programmes in these countries/regions have a predominance of informal or non-formal modes of learning. Particularly, interest classes were most welcomed by elder learners.

The above provides a general overview of the four countries/regions in terms of the context of promoting elder learning. In the second part of this chapter, the specific pattern of elder learning in the four countries/regions will be described, making reference to their respective socio-historical context.

China

Overview of the Development of Lifelong Learning for the Elderly in China

As mentioned in the introductory section, China places high emphasis on protecting and promoting the rights and interests of the elderly people. There are specific statutory provisions serving such a purpose. The China National Committee on Ageing is the body within the Central Government vested with the responsibility to promoting elderly welfare. With respect to elderly learning, Article 31 of the Law on Protection of the Rights and Interests of the Elderly stipulates that the elderly have the right to receive continuing education. In 1994, the National Seven-Year Development Plan of the Work on Aging was worked out by the collaborative efforts of ten ministries of the Central Government. This Plan is to mobilize and require the local governments at all levels to work out a development plan for the education of the elderly (Xiao 2000). Governments at various levels provide support to promoting elder lifelong learning by funding in the form of seed money or a lump-sum subsidy (Lai et al. 1995), premises and guidelines for management. There are also collaborative efforts among various government departments, e.g. Committees for the Elderly at various levels, different organizations (including the government's Education Department, Employment and Manpower Department, Finance Department and so on) in support of such endeavours. Grounded upon the societal norm of respecting and caring for the elderly, there is also good community partnership between public and private sectors, in which enterprises, working units, community organizations and elderly groups join efforts in providing support to elderly education, which could involve the provision of funding, staff, venues and equipment.

Similar to the trend of marketization in the economy, as well as the 'socialization of social welfare' policy, the Chinese government has also adopted a 'community-based' approach in developing its elder-learning projects. It is, in fact, also congruent with the Communist Party's conventional 'grassroots' approach in mass mobilization, especially with its pervasive and extensive network of local level party organizations. Thus, as Wolff (2008) suggested, China is moving from a national-, organization- and enterprise-based system to a community-based system or from a wholly publicly financed system to a system encouraging mixed public and private financing in implementing elder learning. This approach has the merit of providing courses that can better fit the needs of older persons in their respective communities, and educational opportunities are more easily accessible to the elderly. It can also mobilize local resources, including teaching staff, venue and funding (Lui et al. 2002).

At the community level, there are three layers of elderly learning organizations or units: at the community, street and residents' committee levels, respectively. The programmes may involve social-recreational, sport and cultural activities as well as those that promote the elderly people's contribution to the community, for instance, in promoting older persons' assistance and care to younger people. It is primarily based on the government's endorsement and promulgation of the traditional Chinese proverb that says, 'Elderly could serve the community'. It is believed that the elderly people have life wisdom accumulated through their rich life experiences, and thus, their potential in transmitting their knowledge and wisdom to the next generation should be capitalized. For instance, the curriculum of elder learning programmes is designed with a view to enhancing and recognizing the elderly people's contribution to the family in such aspects as handling household chores and attending to children as well as their contribution to society by way of working in small businesses or engaging in civic affairs. To illustrate, as reported by the Beijing Retired People Association, more than 30,000 older persons returned to work in 6,000 organizations after re-training in the period 1986–1996 (Ma 1998). These community-based projects are by and large the mainstream of elder learning initiatives in China, while Senior University or U3A only constitutes a minority of some 2% (Chen 2006).

The first U3A was set up by the Red Cross in Shandong in 1983, followed by many others in other major Chinese cities. This was an initiative by the Red Cross as follow-up action and lobbying after an elderly conference in Vienna in July 1982 (Lai et al. 1995). In China, only those institutes that are recognized by the relevant education ministries or departments in achieving a designated level of educational standard could be named as 'university'. However, Senior's University is an exception to this, which reveals the Chinese government's intent to promote elder learning with a more liberal stance. There is generally no formal system for approving the curriculum, and the teachers who are mostly older persons can decide the curriculum in consultation with the students and based on their expertise (Lui et al. 2002). In 1988, the China Association of Universities for the Aged (CAUA) was formed to provide a platform for various U3As to have collaboration and exchanges at the national level. The CAUA also cooperates with the Central Radio/TV University to offer courses and with national publishers to publish textbooks (Thompson 2002). From then onwards, there has been spectacular growth in both the numbers of elderly universities/colleges and students enrolled over the years: 71 and 30,000, respectively, in 1985; 289 and 100,000 in 1987; and 3,100 and 300,000 in 1991 (Lai et al. 1995). Furthermore, as in 2006, there were some 26,000 U3As with some 2.3 million elderly student enrolments (Chen 2006). In fact, China has the world's largest number of U3As (Thompson 2002). Currently, such developments have already reached the provincial, municipal, county, community and village levels. From its initial inception, most of the participants were retired cadres, senior officials or retirees from state-owned enterprises. This is particularly so as China has a legacy of planned economy before liberalization in the early 1980s, where work units would provide various kinds of welfare to their employees and retirees, including post-retirement recreation and education. However, the most recent development has enabled a more inclusive pattern of enrolment where ordinary senior citizens can also be benefited, especially with the proliferation of community-based, rather than work-unit-based, welfare provision.

Culminating from the 1990s, radio and television broadcasting has been added on to elder learning programmes. The first of this kind, the Shanghai Air Elderly University was founded in October 1995 and was then followed in 1999 by the Shanghai Web-based Elderly University. Such a development is essentially based on the rapid development in information technologies engendered by China's gathering momentum in economic prosperity. The Air University best serves older persons who are not mobile or who are living in remote areas where qualified teachers are lacking through broadcasting educational programmes on television.

Problems and Prospects

The promotion of elder learning has gradually gathered momentum both at the governmental and community levels. However, though there has already been some 30 years of development, there is yet no national legislation governing the implementation of elder learning in China. It was only in 2002 that the city of Tientsin enacted a local ordinance that stipulates the municipal government's responsibility in overseeing, regulating and supporting elder learning. There may be the urgent need to devise a statutory and regulatory regime in further protecting the rights of elder learners and regulating the quality and provision of elder service providers.

On the other hand, since China is such a huge country with a tremendous population as well as a looming large ageing population, it is quite unconceivable that the government could shoulder all the responsibilities in promoting and providing elder learning opportunities. It thus has to tap into the momentum and resources from the private sector – both the market and the growing body of non-profit organizations – to supplement the promotion of elder learning. In fact, there has already been some positive signs in this direction: As estimated by Holford et al. (1998), there were some 5,000 elderly institutes in 1994 in China that were sponsored by private foundations.

There is also stark contrast between the urban and rural regions in the development of elder learning. The urban areas excel over their rural counterparts in having more older persons participating in elderly learning activities, and a higher level of educational quality. While elder learning institutes and initiatives in the urban areas may promote older persons' self-development and adopt non-instrumental orientation, those found in the rural areas are more pragmatic and instrumental and are related to daily livelihood, for instance, in enhancing technical competence of rural elders engaging in agrarian production. This pragmatic stance adopted by China in its promotion of elder learning was noted as somewhat different from that of its western counterparts, like Finland, where elderly education is mainly taken as a means to enhance older persons' adaptability, reduce their dependency and thus improve the quality of their life (Lui et al. 2002). Nonetheless, there could be possible developments that could induce gradual changes to this pattern. For instance, though the rural population still constitutes a considerable portion (to the extent of 60%) in the entire population, such a proportion, in fact, has been diminishing against the background of increasing urbanization all over China. Moreover, with the gradual improvement in literacy and financial capacities of the future cohort of seniors, there could be a larger market for personal development and leisure pursuits, rather than mere pragmatic concerns, in the elder learning activities.

Hong Kong

Overview of the Development of Lifelong Learning for the Elderly in Hong Kong

In Hong Kong, the origin of lifelong learning for older people could be traced back to the eighties when learning opportunities were mainly provided by social service centres for the elderly. Courses offered were not credit-based (Zhang and Ha 2001) and were mostly leisure or recreational in nature. At the beginning, a non-formal approach was adopted (Lee and Chan 2002) that provided structured learning experiences without formal assessment or credentialing (Hamil-Luker and Uhlenberg 2002).

It could be postulated that elder learning has not been a priority for the government both before and after the 1997 handover. It was only when the Elderly Commission was set up in 1997, which in itself was a deliberate move of the inaugural administration to show its embracement of traditional Chinese virtue and cultural normative order (of respecting the elderly), that the Commission was given the mandate to attend to various elderly policy domains. It was thus the Commission that had recognized the significance of lifelong learning for the elders and launched the 'Opportunities for the Elderly Project'. Subsequently in 1999, the then Chief Executive proclaimed such concepts as 'Learning for Life', 'Learning through Life' and 'Successful Ageing', which gave impetus for the promotion of lifelong learning for the elderly (Lui et al. 2002). In 2001, the Hong Kong Jockey Club Charities Trust provided a HK$21-million (about US$2.7 million) grant to support the Elderly Commission to launch the 3-year Community Partnership Scheme to support innovative projects and education programmes that promote healthy ageing in the community.

The profile of participants in lifelong learning in Hong Kong displays some special features. It was found that the males, the old-old and the uneducated were the least likely to participate. On the other hand, those having a higher prior educational level were even more prone to be active participants. Furthermore, socio-economic variables like age, gender, prior educational level, marital status, employment and status and participation in other activities (e.g. community groups, religious groups and volunteer services) were also found to be related to older people's participation in tertiary education (Hong Kong Council of Social Service 2002). With respect to motivation to learning, a local study found that expressive motivation prevailed over instrumental motivation among the elder learners. Nonetheless, those with higher educational attainment held both instrumental and expressive motivations in their participation in lifelong learning activities (Leung et al. 2006). A postgraduate student's study revealed that all the respondents interviewed expressed their wish to accomplish the dream of studying in the university as they did not have this chance when they were young and their families did not have the means to afford their education (Lam 2009). This aptly illustrates the incidence of 'compensatory' motive sustaining the elders' effort in participating lifelong learning.

Lifelong Learning (LLL) Programmes for the Elderly in Hong Kong

There are a variety of LLL programmes in Hong Kong: classroom learning, radio broadcasting and Internet online learning, formal education, travel learning, elder academy and U3A; among them, classroom learning is the most common type.

1. *Classroom learning.* It originated in the 1980s from the interest classes organized by elderly centres at the district and neighbourhood levels. Such classes may include Chinese literacy, simple English, dancing and the like. It should be

recognized that since many of these centres are located in public housing estates where the operating NGOs can tap on the benefit of lower rents charged by the government as a gesture of support to welfare services, the membership of these centres tends to be rather skewed towards those elderly coming from relatively lower socio-economic background, e.g. having lower education and financial means. Thus many of these classes are designed and organized by the professional social workers and delivered by hired or volunteer instructors. This is to be contrasted to the model of U3A that capitalizes on the elder learners' own initiatives.

2. *Radio college for the elderly.* The Hong Kong government operates a radio (and television) broadcasting department that disseminates government information and promotes public education, namely, the Radio Television Hong Kong (RTHK). Since 1999, the RTHK designates a specific channel named 'Radio 5' that operates the Radio College for the Elderly that provides classes and tutorial workshops for the elderly audience.
3. *Online learning.* The merit of online learning is that it provides universal and easy access at any time and any place, without the problems of having a quota, unavailability of venue or expensive rental costs. Furthermore, even frail and home-bound elders can also have the opportunity to participate in lifelong learning. However, the possible problem of the digital divide is putting older persons at a disadvantage in accessing information and services, and thus, they suffer from social exclusion. For instance, it was reported that in Hong Kong, in 2006, senior citizens lagged behind in Internet utilization the most when compared with other major disadvantaged groups, including single parents, children of low-income households, new migrants, female homemakers and persons with disabilities and chronic illnesses (Wong et al. 2009). In addition, only about 10% of Hong Kong's elders are computer literate and have access to computers (Hong Kong SAR Government, Census and Statistics Department 2009). In the era of 'information society', the digital divide may jeopardize social inclusion of older persons and thus their dignity. Recently, there are efforts by the government's Elderly Commission and NGOs in promoting elderly people's utilization and mastery of computer skills by providing training courses at schools and elderly centres.
4. *Learning programmes built in the formal educational system.* Although the Hong Kong government has deployed substantial resources in education, such efforts are nearly entirely targeting the youth population. The older people are practically excluded from the formal education system in Hong Kong. Thus, it is a particularly bold attempt by a local university, Lingnan University, in collaboration with a local NGO, the Hong Kong Society for the Aged (SAGE), to launch in 2002 an associate degree programme majoring in Applied Gerontology for people above 50 years old. The programme has a special nomenclature, that of 'Dream for University Education', to provide older adults beyond the age of 50 a chance to study at a university, as this really constitutes a 'dream' for many of those who had lost such a chance during their early years due to poverty, war and other circumstances. The programme does not require the older adults to meet certain academic eligibility criteria, as distinct from other associate degree

programmes offered in the tertiary institutes or the formal education system in Hong Kong. One of the special features of the programme is to admit also ordinary school-leavers who are at their late teens. Thus, there is a natural mix of students of different ages, thus promoting inter-generational contact. The curriculum is to provide students with a better understanding of the challenges and opportunities in an ageing society. Apart from the conventional university mode of lectures and tutorials, a special feature of the programme is to arrange students to have practicum in elderly services organizations to capitalize on experiential learning. Interviews with the adult students revealed that they had achieved a great deal of satisfaction in the learning process and regained a sense of self-efficacy and worth (Lam 2009).

5. *Elderhostel.* With the gradual improvement in the socio-economic status of some elderly people in Hong Kong, there is an increasing trend that older people engage more in travel, both local and overseas. Thus, recently, some NGOs have started organizing 'Elderhostels', which is modelled after the 'Youth Hostel' movement in the USA in particular. Elderhostels may 'combine the romance of travel to interesting places with the opportunity to learn and socialize with interesting peers' (Lamdin and Fugate 1997:103). It is anticipated that with the progression of the baby boomers into their retirement stage, there could be considerable development in this mode of elder learning, given the improved health, education and financial resources.
6. *Elder academy.* As an initiative to promote elder learning, the government and the Elderly Commission in 2007 jointly launched the Elder Academy Scheme, which aims to encourage elders to continue learning. In the scheme, local primary and secondary school and welfare organizations serve as sponsoring bodies to run 'elder academies' in which elderly people have the chance to work and interact with young students, thus promoting inter-generational harmony and cross-sectoral collaboration. The aims of the scheme, according to the Elderly Commission, are to promote continuous learning and encourage elders to widen their social networks, maintain physical and mental well-being and foster a sense of worth while acquiring knowledge (Elderly Commission 2010). More specific objectives include the following: to promote lifelong learning, to maintain healthy physical and mental well-being, to realize the objective of fostering a sense of worthiness in elders, to optimize existing resources, to promote harmony between the elders and the young, to strengthen civic education and to promote cross-sectoral harmony (ibid). As in 2010, there were more than 100 elder academies established in primary, secondary and tertiary education institutions.
7. *U3A development.* In 2006, the U3A Network was launched with the initiation from the Hong Kong Council of Social Service (HKCSS), which was supported by Hong Kong Electric Centenary Trust (HKECT). The HKCSS and HKECT also provide support in the management of the U3A centres and assist in promotion. The Trust provides seed money to affiliated members of the HKCSS. Such agencies should set up a 'U3A Center' and recruit at least 12 U3A members to form a management committee and to organize ten courses in two seasons, benefiting at least 120 participants. The target participants are those aged 50 and

above, in view of catering for those who have early retirement and those housewives who have relinquished their household duties. Participants are encouraged to teach and manage their respective U3A learning centres so as to promote lifelong learning and volunteerism in serving the community. The project operates on a model of emphasizing four 'self' aspects, namely, 'self-initiating, self-managing, self-teaching and self-learning'. Most U3As are operated on a self-financed basis and are manned only by elderly volunteers with no paid staff. However, some of them affiliate to some local NGOs that operate elderly services, e.g. the elderly centres at district and neighbourhood levels. There are three streams of courses offered, namely, 'knowledge-based', 'interest-based' and 'self-enhancement'.

There are also obstacles confronting the U3A initiatives in Hong Kong. Given that land and house prices and rents in Hong Kong are spectacularly high, the U3As may not be able to afford expensive rental costs and so have to rely on the venues provided by the social service centres to which they affiliate. In turn, these elderly service NGOs also rely on the government's provision of low-rented venues in public rental housing estates in the form of 'welfare premise'. Alternatively, the Open University of Hong Kong supports the U3A initiative by providing venues for the participants.

Problems and Prospects

At its current stage, elder learning in general is still in its embryonic stage. It is probably due to the fact that the current cohort of elderly people in Hong Kong is marked by a substantial portion of low socio-economic status and has low (or even no) literacy, unsatisfactory financial security and even physical limitations due to frailty and poor health. It is anticipated that, with the coming cohort of elders having more favourable resource endowment in various aspects, health, finance, education, the further development of elderly learning could be remarkable.

Although there is possibly a positive scenario for the further development of elderly education, there are still problems and hurdles to work through. For instance, the government has not yet devised comprehensive policy and a plan to promote elderly lifelong learning. Worse still, there appears to be an inherent ageist stance among government officials in depriving elderly people of their fair share of support in participating in education. The government has instituted the Continuous Education Fund (CEF) that is supposed to support adults to pursue continuing education for personal and professional development. However, it apparently has a skewed emphasis on career or occupational training, as the eligible age range is capped at 65. It practically denies those senior citizens beyond this age their right to receive this subsidy. Though the Hong Kong government has invested a lot in education with the policy domain of education ranked top in the government's annual recurrent expenses, it is largely for the formal education for young people, but not the elders.

Taiwan

Overview of the Development of Lifelong Learning for the Elderly in Taiwan

The origin of elder learning in Taiwan could be traced back to the establishment of the first 'Evergreen Academy' in the city of Kaohsiung in 1982 by the municipal Social Affairs Bureau in collaboration with the Young Women's Christian Association. Subsequently, the Air University was first set up in 1985. In fact, the promotion of elder learning could be seen as one of the strategies of the Taiwan government in promoting active ageing. In order to promote senior citizens' active participation in society, there are policies and programmes that serve such a purpose, including the provision of discounts for elders in transportation, access to facilities and activities. There is also a special 'senior citizens manpower bank' that helps to facilitate elders engaging in paid work or volunteer services. The Ministry of Interior would designate special budgets for setting up senior citizens' facilities at the county and village levels. In 1990, the Ministry of Education (MoE) had already included the aspect of elder learning in its policy initiatives on social learning. Such measures included the provision of training for elders who looked for re-employment; radio broadcasting; holding series of talks for retirement protection; and curriculum design for elder learning. In the following year of 1991, the MoE designated the 5-year Elder Learning Implementation Plan. The Plan specifies three specific objectives: firstly, to enable elders to have better adjustment to life transitions and achieve self-actualization through re-education and re-socializing; secondly, to assist those elders who have the motivation to work to have re-training and then re-employment so as to capitalize on their rich life experience and talents; and thirdly, to promote traditional Chinese cultural value of respecting the elders by developing the elders' physical, psychological and spiritual health and by expanding the life circle. The scope of this elder learning programme includes five domains, namely, basic education, professional skills, health, leisure and inter-generational relationship. These curricula are delivered through radio and television broadcast as well as centre-based (including NGOs, schools and elderly centres) programmes.

The MoE, based upon the accomplishments of the first 5-year programme plan, started its 1996 programme plan to provide financial support to set up community lifelong learning centres at public primary and secondary schools. Two initiatives are particularly relevant to senior citizens. Firstly, elder learning centres are set up within schools that recruit volunteers aged 50 or above to arrange programmes and activities for elderly community members to participate in learning and social activities. Special effort would be made to recruit elderly volunteers who can serve as teachers or instructors for programme participants. Another innovative project is the setting up of school-based 'community toys workshop' in which elder volunteers are recruited to help repair toys for primary school students. This promotes the intergenerational contact between senior citizens and children and could enhance the self-esteem and confidence of elders who have conventionally been regarded as losing their competence and social functionality. Special mention should be made of the care and prudence given by the MOE officials in the design of such elder learning and activity facilities: All these centres are well placed in classrooms that are near to toilets, which cater for the need of elderly people who might have a bladder control problem.

Furthermore, the MoE designated 1998 as the Year of Lifelong Learning and published the White Paper on 'Heading Towards Learning Society'. Most significantly, the government enacted the Act on Lifelong Learning in 2002, which provides statutory protection for lifelong learning for the people. The MoE promulgated the Senior Education Policy White Paper in 2006, which further buttresses the protection of senior citizens' right to lifelong learning. The policy paper was targeted at solving the problems of the development of senior education in Taiwan. Such problems include the lack of proper regulations and an integrated mechanism in promoting the multi-faceted system, no secured assurance on the funding for promotion, low motivation in participation found in the public, lack of innovations of the elderly courses curriculums, teaching materials and teaching methods, lack of designated venue for the elderly education in the community, inadequate professional training provided for the instructors and the lack of support for research on elderly education (MoE 2006). Later in 2008, the MoE launched the plan for establishing elder learning resource centres at the county and town levels. It also promoted the setting up of lifelong learning centres for senior citizens at universities. Such centres provide free-of-charge short-stay (i.e. 5 days) arrangement for elderly to engage in learning activities. Such an approach, which is also prevalent in other advanced economies, capitalizes on the existing resources of the universities in academic expertise, venue and facilities. By 2009, there were 28 universities that operated such lifelong learning centres.

According to the statistics of the Ministry of Interior, as at the year 2000, there were 303 Evergreen Centres (Taiwan Ministry of Interior 2003). On the other hand, the 2001 figures from the National Open University reveal that there were some 1,196 senior citizens aged 60 or above attending courses (National Open University 2001). In the year 2009, there were 23,465 classes with 592,932 participants throughout the various counties and cities in Taiwan (Ministry of Education of Taiwan 2010). Regarding the profile of elderly participants in the elder learning activities, senior-academic–related organizations (e.g. Evergreen Academy and Elderly University that are mainly located in urbanized regions) had the highest rate of participation: 24.8%; social educational organizations (including culture centres, libraries, China Youth Corps, etc.) stood as the second: 20.9%; the last were senior clubs: 16.3%.

Problems and Prospects

The evolution of elder learning in Taiwan has undergone different stages. According to Chen (2009), there could be four phases. The first dates back to post-1949–1970 when remedial education was provided to the elderly. The second stage was marked by 'radio broadcasted education' and promotion by universities in the period 1971–1980. In the third stage, between 1981 and 2005, it was the development of 'Evergreen Academy' or 'Elder University'. Most recently, the fourth phase witnessed the promulgation of the Senior Education Policy White Paper in 2006 and the introduction of 'Elder Learning Centres' in 2008. Alternatively, it could be viewed as having been a gradual evolution from the initiation stage in which elder learning was organized by religious bodies. Later with the introduction of the law on elderly welfare, elder learning took on a welfare orientation, as most senior citizen universities and elder learning institutes were operated by welfare departments of the county and municipal governments. Subsequently, in the 1990s, lifelong learning was heralded as the leading orientation. In Wang's (2007 framework, cited in Chen 2009), it could be framed as undergoing the stages of initiation and then welfare and lastly of intervention from education policies. Thus, there is considerable prospect of development with the government's dedicated commitment and resource input.

Most recently, there is also a recent change in the approach adopted by the government. There appears to be an emerging trend where elder lifelong learning would progress towards a 'bottom-up' or 'community approach' in which the government would 'contract out' such programmes and activities to civic organizations, promoting public–private collaboration and partnership. In addition, it also promotes user-pay and local (community) governance or management that capitalizes on the ownership, independence and initiatives of local organizations. This could be seen as a strategy of promoting the development of civic society (Chen 2009).

Similar to other countries and places, lifelong learning in Taiwan is also implemented in formal, informal and non-formal contexts. Formal learning involves the universities and academies, while informal and non-formal ones are operated at community and cultural centres. Elder learning is currently implemented by different sectors and organizations. The Air University and compensatory education are operated by the government's education departments; the Evergreen Centre and other elderly social centres are operated by the government welfare departments, while the community colleges and senior citizen universities are managed by religious or non-government non-profit organizations (Chen 2009). On the whole, senior learning programmes are mainly run by NGOs and social welfare departments at various levels, which are much more active than education departments of the government. There may be the need to have better integration and synergy between these various sectors and organizations in the provision of elder lifelong learning programmes.

However, there are challenges confronting the development of elder learning in Taiwan. The government has recognized that though there were numerous elderly participants, there has also been considerable duplication of membership without much new enrolment. This had resulted in having no significant breakthrough and growth in the field of senior education (The Ministry of Education 2006). Wu (1997) suggested that there are six main problems confronting the development of elder learning in Taiwan, namely, the lack of designated organization for promotion, inadequacy in legal framework, low participation rate among elders, insufficient manpower infrastructure, low motivation among teachers and inadequate budgets and publicity. However, the fundamental issue lies in the inadequate integration of efforts between the welfare and education departments of the government.

Singapore

Overview of the Development of Lifelong Learning for the Elderly in Singapore

The Singaporean government is highly cognizant of the small size of the country and economy amidst the increasingly competitive globalized world context. Thus, it has placed high emphasis and investment on education, the expenditure of which ranks top. In promoting the competitiveness of its workforce, the government has promoted lifelong learning for its whole population, including the senior citizens. Singapore's approach to lifelong learning is pragmatic and rational and serves as one of the economic drivers to enhance the country's competitiveness as well as a means to counteract unemployment (Kumar 2004). The Ministry of Manpower is vested with the authority and responsibility of promoting lifelong learning since 2000. However, probably due to the relatively small size of its population, coupled with the upcoming trend and challenges of an ageing population, the focus of promoting lifelong learning has been placed on enhancing people's employability. In this regard, the target population of such programmes is those who are less skilled and have lower educational attainment. The Singapore Workforce Development Agency (WDA), which was set up in 2003, also has the function of providing retraining and job placement for senior citizens. Its mission is to 'enhance the employability and competitiveness of all in the workforce, young and old from rank-and-file to professionals, managers and executives' (Singapore Workforce Development Agency 2010). The Singaporean government provides basic social infrastructure to promote learning among the public. In this vein, public libraries are located within public housing estates and are thus easily accessible to the public, as more than 90% of the Singaporean population lives in government for-sale and rental housing estates. As an incentive for promoting people's active engagement in lifelong learning, the government provides Lifelong Learner Awards to give recognition to participants who have outstanding performance and positive learning attitudes. These awardees would then serve as Learning Ambassadors to help promote and propagate lifelong learning among the general public. The government also organizes the Singapore Learning Festival to enhance the citizens' identification, with the goal of lifelong learning and of employability (Ministry of Manpower 2003).

With respect to elder learning, public libraries' facilities are designed to be elder friendly. For instance, lifts and access ramps are provided for people in a wheelchair, including elders. In more subtle ways, the book shelves and height of placement of books are specially designed and arranged to enable seniors' easy reach to the books. The government's Committee on Ageing Issues encourages the library to further enhance elder-friendliness by providing books with large prints and audiovisual materials that may be more appropriate for elders with lower educational attainment or literacy. The Committee also encourages the universities and polytechnics to provide more learning opportunities to seniors. These could involve courses that are short-term and not to be examined formally, to avoid the stress induced to the elder learners. Alternatively, the universities may allow seniors to attend their normal lectures and seminars and to access course curriculum and materials free of charge. With such opportunities, elder people could be able to have the incentive and support to form into home-based study groups in their pursuit of university-based learning. For instance, the National University of Singapore Extension has its Centre for Lifelong Learning that offers courses in language, literature and culture for elderly people.

Apart from government efforts, community organizations also organize courses for seniors. For example, Marine Parade Family Service Centre has taken the initiative to operate 'YAH! Community College',, which offers courses for elders to acquire information and communication technology and develop life skills. In such community colleges, elder people aged 55 and above can enrol in lifelong learning courses that may lead to the award of a certificate. The Active Ageing Academy (AAA) is the first U3A type of elderly learning institute in Singapore. It offers a 6-month programme on basic counselling skills and knowledge of third-age wellness, leading to a double certification for participants. As there is a sizeable Chinese population among the elderly in Singapore, the programme is conducted in Mandarin. The programme operates with conventional interactive classroom learning as well as field trips and experiential service learning through community projects. Such a programme contributes to promoting active ageing of seniors.

Problems and Prospects

A study (Tan 2010) revealed that Singaporean seniors were not as active as desired in participating in elder learning programmes. Specifically, they were less interested in job- or career-related courses than in leisure- or hobby-related courses of elder learning. It was suggested that, given Singapore's shortage of manpower, seniors should be encouraged to stay employable and to be employed longer. Thus, elder learning programmes should promote job- or career-related courses to the elderly people. There may be the need to segment the market whereby job- or career-related courses are to be offered to younger seniors and non-job- or career-related courses to older seniors. In this regard, there are issues that should be attended to in order to boost their participation rates, including the enhancement of convenience, accessibility, affordability and practical content relating to courses and connectedness in regard to learning environment (Tan 2010).

Summary and Concluding Remarks

With reference to the framework formulated by Aspin and Chapman (2007), lifelong learning policy in different countries can be categorized, according to the targets of the recipients and the goals of education, into four major categories. Firstly, the compensatory education model is to rectify the social inequalities precipitated in the formal education system. Secondly, the continuing vocational training model aims at enhancing competence of the general or specific population in their occupations. Thirdly, the social innovation model helps to promote socio-economic development. Fourthly, the leisure-oriented model provides learning activities premised on leisure and social recreational motivations. As revealed in the four countries/regions examined in this chapter, there are divergences of strategies adopted by different governments in their respective elder learning policies. The above review helps to provide a spectrum of modalities and programmes that serve as reference for different countries in their effort in promoting elder learning. All in all, given that it is practically inevitable for all developed countries to face up to the challenges posed by an increasingly ageing population, governments of these countries should be aware of the potential magnitude of the problems, as well as the latent resources, embedded in a large and increasing elderly population. The promotion of elder learning should not be the sole responsibility of governments alone, but should be shared by the larger community in which respect for elders should form the groundwork. Age discrimination, which entails negative stereotypes against elderly people as inept for learning or change, should be reduced, if not eradicated. The senior citizens, no matter from which walks of life, whether having or not previous educational attainment, as far as possible, should engage themselves actively in lifelong learning activities because it has been confirmed by research findings that continued learning is important for active ageing and that active ageing is also the key to adding life to years, it is thus desirable and imperative indeed for governments all over the world to promote lifelong learning for their older people, as one of the strategies in tackling the challenges of an ageing population.

References

Aspin, D. N., & Chapman, J. D. (2007). Lifelong learning: Concepts and conceptions. In D. N. Aspin (Ed.), *Philosophical perspectives on lifelong learning*. Dordrecht: Springer.

Boulton-Lewis, G. M., Buys, L., & Lovie-Kitchin, J. (2006). Learning and active aging. *Educational Gerontology, 32*(4), 271–282.

Chen, N. L. (2006, November 3–4). *A reflection on the development of elder learning in China.* Paper presented at 2006 East Asia Elder Learning Strategies Seminar. Taipei.

Chen, Y. J. (2009, October). *Historical development and mode of operation of Elder Universities in Taiwan.* Paper presented at Forum on Elder Universities, Shanghai, China.

Chui, E. (2007). Changing norms and pragmatics of co-residence in East Asian countries. *International Journal of Sociology of the Family, 33*(1), 1–24.

Committee on Ageing Issues, Singapore Government. (2006). *Report on the ageing population, Five-year masterplan*. Singapore. Retrieved May 23, 2010, from http://www.mcys.gov.sg/successful_ageing/report/CAI_report.pdf

Directorate-General of Budget, Taiwan. (2010). Accounting and statistics, executive Yuan, Taiwan. *2009 Analysis of Final Central Government Accounts* [in Chinese]. Retrieved May 21, 2010, from http://www.dgbas.gov.tw/ct.asp?xItem=26671&CtNode=5196&mp=1

Elderly Commission, Hong Kong. (2010). http://www.elderlycommission.gov.hk/

Glendenning, F. (2001). Education for older adults. *International Journal of Lifelong Education, 20*(1/2), 63–70.

Hamil-Luker, J., & Uhlenberg, P. (2002). Later life education in the 1990s: Increasing involvement and continuing disparity. *Journals of Gerontology Series B: Psychological Sciences and Social Sciences, 57B*, 324–332.

Holford, J., Jarvis, P., & Griffin, C. (Eds.). (1998). *International perspectives on lifelong learning*. London: Kogan Page.

Holliday, I. (2000). Productivist welfare capitalism: Social policy in East Asia. *Political Studies, 48*, 706–723.

Hong Kong Council of Social Service. (2002). *Learning needs and preferences of members of multi-service members for elderly and social centres for elderly* (Final Report Hong Kong). Hong Kong: The Hong Kong Council of Social Service.

Hong Kong SAR Government. (2010). Summary of expenditure estimates. *The Budget 2010–11*. Retrieved from http://www.budget.gov.hk/2010/eng/pdf/sum_exp_e.pdf

Hong Kong SAR Government. Census and Statistics Department. (2009). *Thematic Household Survey Report No. 43. Information Technology Usage and Penetration.* Hong Kong: Hong Kong SAR Government. Census and Statistics Department.

Kim, A., & Merriam, S. B. (2004). Motivations for learning among older adults in a learning in retirement institute. *Educational Gerontology, 30*, 441–455.

Kumar, P. (2004). Lifelong learning in Singapore: Where are we now? *International Journal of Lifelong Education, 23*(6), 559–568.

Lai, S. M., Tse, A. P., & Tang, W. L. (1995). Elderly education in mainland China. *Adult education in China* (pp. 427–447). China: Kao Ah Fook Man Publisher, Beijing.

Lam, F. Y. Y. (2009). *A study of the tertiary education experience of older adults in Hong Kong*. Unpublished thesis. The University of Hong Kong, Pokfulam.

Lamdin, L., & Fugate, M. (1997). *Elderlearning: New frontier in an aging society. American Council on Education Series on Higher Education*. Phoenix: Oryx.

Lee, W. O. (1996). The cultural context for Chinese learners: Conceptions of learning in the Confucian tradition. In D. Watkins & J. Biggs (Eds.), *The Chinese learner: Cultural, psychological and contextual influences* (pp. 25–41). Melbourne/Hong Kong: Hong Kong Cooperative Education Research Centre/The Australian Council for Educational Research.

Lee, P. W. & Chan, K. M. (2002, March 16). *Development of lifelong learning among Hong Kong new generative elderly: Abstract of final research report* [In Chinese]. Paper presented at the Hong Kong Young Women Christian Association, Hong Kong.

Leung, A., Lui, Y. H., & Chi, I. (2006). Later life learning experience among Chinese elderly in Hong Kong. *Gerontology & Geriatrics Education, 26*(2), 1–15.

Lui, Y. H., Leung, A., & Jegede, O. J. (2002). *Research report on overseas experience in providing continuing education for older persons*. Hong Kong: The Open University of Hong Kong.

Ma, S. P. (1998). *Establishment of lifelong education system: Practice and research on Beijing adult education* [In Chinese]. Hong Kong: People Educational Publisher.

Ministry of Education of Taiwan. (2010). *Senior Education*. Retrieved April 10, 2010, from http://moe.senioredu.moe.gov.tw/front/bin/ptdetail.phtml?Part=09120004&Category=68

Ministry of Finance, People's Republic of China. (2010). *Report on the implementation of the 2009 and 2010 central and local budgets*. Retrieved May 21, 2010, from http://www.mof.gov.cn/zhengwuxinxi/caizhengxinwen/201003/t20100316_276816.html

Ministry of Manpower, Singapore Government. (2003). *The Singapore Learning Festival Pushes Message on Lifelong Learning for Employability*. Retrieved May 12, 2007, from http://www.

mom.gov.sg/publish/momportal/en/press_room/press_releases/2003/20031114-TheSingaporeLearningFestivalPushesMessageOnLifelongLearningForEmployability.html

National Open University. Taiwan. (2001). *Statistics report of the student distribution 1997–2001*. Retrieved May 27, 2010, from http://www.nou.edu.tw/~research/news/data_05_86-90_S06.htm

Population Reference Bureau. (2009). *Population Age 65+(%). PRB 2009 World Population Data Sheet*. Retrieved from http://www.prb.org/Datafinder/Topic/Bar.aspx?sort=v&order=d&variable=119

Poston, D. L., Jr., & Duan, C. C. (2000). The current and projected distribution of the elderly and eldercare in the People's Republic of China. *Journal of Family Issues, 21*, 714–732.

Ramesh, M. (2004). *Social policy in East and Southeast Asia: Education, health housing and income maintenance*. London: Routledge-Curzon.

Singapore Department of Statistics. (2010). *Monthly Digest of Statistics Singapore*. Retrieved February 2010, from http://www.singstat.gov.sg/pubn/reference/mdsfeb10.pdf

Singapore Ministry of Community Development and Sports. (2001). Eldercare Master Plan (FY2001 to FY2005).

Singapore Workforce Development Agency. (2010). About WDA, Our Vision & Mission. Retrieved May 23, 2010, from http://app2.wda.gov.sg/web/Contents/Contents.aspx?ContId=8

Taiwan Ministry of Interior, Department of Statistics. (2003). *Social data*. Retrieved from http://www.moi.gov.tw/stat/english/download.asp

Taiwan Ministry of Interior, Social Service Bureau. (2010). Retrieved from http://sowf.moi.gov.tw/04/01.htm

Tan, E. S. (2010). *MCYS Survey on the learning needs of senior in Singapore*. Singapore: Council for Third Age. Retrieved March 15, 2010, from http://www.c3a.org.sg/images/pdf/MCYS%20Learning%20Needs%20Survey_Full%20Report.pdf.

Tang, K. L. (2000). *Social welfare development in East Asia*. Basingstoke: Palgrave.

The Ministry of Education. (2006). *Action of learning society integrated planning research: Planning of Senior Education*. Retrieved March 5, 2010, from http://moe.senioredu.moe.gov.tw/front/bin/ptlist.phtml?Category=63

Thompson, J. (2002). *The Amazing University of the Third Age in China today*. Retrieved March 4, 2010, from http://worldu3a.org/resources/u3a-china.htm

Wang, F. S. (2007). Elder learning in Taiwan. In F. S. Wang (Ed.), *Elder learning: International review* (pp. 29–49). Taipei: Wunan.

Withnall, A. (2006). Exploring influences on later life learning. *International Journal of Lifelong Education, 25*(1), 29–49.

Wolff, L. (2008). *Lifelong learning for the third age*. Retrieved March 4, 2010, from http://electric.toodoc.com/doc/4035/

Wong, Y. C., Fung, J. Y. C., Law, C. K., Lam, J. C. Y., & Lee, V. (2009). Tackling the digital divide. *British Journal of Social Work, 39*(4), 754–767.

Wu, J. M (1997) *The research of Elder Education in Taiwan*. Retrieved from http://wjm58603.myweb.hinet.net/work.htm

Xiao, C. (2000). China: Lifelong learning and the use of new technology. *TechKnowLogia*. Retrieved March 4, 2010, from http://www.techknowlogia.org/TKL_Articles/PDF/171.pdf

Zhang, W. Y. & Ha, S. (2001). *An investigation into the learning attitude, motivation and preferences of the older adults in Hong Kong*. A paper presented for the 15th Annual Conference of the Asian Association of Open Universities hosted by Indira Gandhi National Open University, New Delhi, India.

Chapter 10
Active Ageing, Active Learning: Elder Learning in Hong Kong

Maureen Tam

The East–West Dichotomous View of Lifelong Learning

Western and Eastern scholarship and learning are often conceived of and described in terms of the Confucian-Western dichotomy (Ryan and Louie 2007). According to Confucian beliefs, lifelong learning is a lifelong effort aimed at forging a morally excellent life and becoming a virtuous person (Kim 2004:117). Learning was conceived by Confucius as 'learning for the sake of the self' as opposed to 'learning for the sake of others'. The latter is said to characterize the instrumental and competition-directed notions of lifelong learning in the West for survival or competitive purposes in a knowledge-based society (Kim 2004:120). However, such contrasting Eastern and Western notions of lifelong learning are considered to be overly simplistic and far from accurate. Chapman et al. (2006) proposed that lifelong learning can be conceptualized as having three over-arching purposes: (1) learning for a more highly skilled work force and a strong economy, (2) learning for a better democracy and an inclusive society, and (3) learning for a more personally rewarding life. The third purpose is congruent with the Confucian notion of lifelong learning as a process of self-betterment, personal growth, and development and may actually be the purpose for learning by elders in all cultures.

Combining the three purposes, learning is considered important and should be continued throughout life, as part of one's personal growth and development and as participation in a democratic society, as well as a contribution to economic growth and development. Implicit in the notion of lifelong learning is the need for all to have equal access to programmes and activities of lifelong learning and the need to

M. Tam (✉)
Department of International Education and Lifelong Learning,
Hong Kong Institute of Education, Tai Po, Hong Kong
e-mail: msltam@ied.edu.hk

G.M. Boulton-Lewis and M. Tam (eds.), *Active Ageing, Active Learning: Issues and Challenges*, Education in the Asia-Pacific Region: Issues, Concerns and Prospects 15,
DOI 10.1007/978-94-007-2111-1_10,

participate fully and freely in such programmes and activities. These general descriptions about lifelong learning should be relevant to older learners, who may however perceive continued learning in older age from their own cultural perspective. In a study that focused on older adults to understand how cultural values shape learning in older adulthood in Malaysia, Merriam and Mohamad (2000) discovered that learning in old age is non-formal and experiential, communal and much of it spiritual or religious in nature. These findings are congruent with the general descriptions that family relationships, the community and spiritual life appear to be much more important with Eastern elderly, reflecting Eastern cultural values of the collective, harmony and spirituality.

There is also a general belief that Chinese or Asian students with a Confucian-heritage cultural (CHC) background are more diligent and highly motivated by achievement. A strong CHC background may influence the way learners conceptualize, approach and engage in learning. Notable research in this area includes the work by Lee about the influence of Confucian-heritage cultures (CHC) on learning (Lee 1996). He asserted that Asian learners are influenced by CHC and therefore have a high regard for education. With a Confucian background, Asian people generally display a positive attitude towards education and are achievement oriented and willing to spend a lot of their free time on studies (Lee 1996:25).

Other cultural value studies have also identified some significant differences in engagement in learning between CHC and Western societies. For example, Lussier (2005) characterized Western culture as individualistic in nature, problem-solving and short-term oriented with a direct and realistic style, whereas the Confucian-influenced societies of East Asia are described as social, family, group and long-term oriented with an indirect communication style and a preference for virtuous behaviour (Lu et al. 2003). Ryan and Louie (2007) have described Western and Asian academic values in binary opposites such as 'deep/surface', 'adversarial/harmonious' and 'independent/dependent'. As Ryan and Louie (2007) have pointed out, however, the descriptions of Western and Asian education systems and scholarship in binary terms do not take into account the complexities and diversity of philosophies of education within and between different educational systems. In the context of elder learning, it is of interest to examine if these general descriptions about Asian and Western learners as younger adults will also be relevant to older learners. There is very little research about the East–West dichotomy in learning, let alone learning for and by older adults. This warrants the need for research to assess the impact of cultural influences on lifelong learning and to examine learning for and by the elderly across different cultural contexts.

Active Ageing and Learning

Research has confirmed that continued learning is important for active ageing (Rowe and Kahn 1999; Ardelt 2000; Glendenning 2001; Jarvis 2001; Boulton-Lewis et al. 2006; Withnall 2006). Schuller et al. (2004) investigated the 'wider benefits of learning' and suggested a framework, in which 12 possible learning benefits are categorized into three forms of capital: human capital (the skills to be deployed), social capital (the set of relationships involved), and identity capital (the personal outlook on life and self-view). In this model, health is conceived of both as an outcome and intermediate factor leading to other benefits of learning. This framework is consistent with similar findings about the positive relationship between health and learning (Ross and Mirowsky 1999; Hammond 2002, 2004; Narushima 2008). In essence, continued learning can help people gain socio-economic, psychological and socio-political resources, all of which in turn lead to a healthier life. In addition to better health, older adults engaged in lifelong learning are found to have positive experiences in at least one of the following areas – enjoyment of life, confidence, self-concept, self-satisfaction and the ability to cope (Dench and Regan 2000). There is, however, limited research evidence to support that engagement in learning or education in early or later life will slow down cognitive decline (Stine-Morrow et al. 2007). Nevertheless, learning keeps older people involved in enjoying and living life fully. It assists in building confidence and self-esteem, slowing down mental decline, building social network, learning new technology and generally keeping them both physically and mentally active and healthy. Brain activity might also be boosted as a result of learning which improves neuroplasticity and supports neural development and new brain cells (Valenzuela 2009). The possible benefits brought about by lifelong learning are important reasons for senior adults to engage in continued learning.

Much of the research into elder learning has been conducted on the issue of needs. McClusky (1971) classified elders' learning needs as coping, expressive, contributive, influence and transcendence. In broader terms, researchers later suggested two main clusters of reasons, or motivations, for elders to engage in learning: expressive and instrumental motivations (O'Connor 1987; Silverstein et al. 2001). Expressive motivation refers to personal development and social relations, while instrumental motivation is related to work, career and skills training. A survey conducted in Hong Kong in 2001 and reported in Leung et al. (2005) revealed that most people aged 55 and above in Hong Kong engaged in learning for five main reasons: to meet people, fill up time, learn something new, make life more meaningful and develop personal interests or hobbies. Generally, these five reasons belong to the category of expressive motivation, as elders are engaging in learning for intrinsic, rather than extrinsic, reasons. Boulton-Lewis et al. (2006) found that older adults have stronger motivation to learn despite the fact that they learn more slowly, need more practice and have varying interests. They also identified a few significant factors for elders to engage in learning, which include being female, having good physical and mental health, level of prior education, living in regional areas, not being retired, and being younger and a higher income earner. The most common reasons older adults gave for continued learning included to exercise the mind, stay mentally stimulated and active, attain certain life goals, and simply never stop learning.

Elder Learning Issues: Needs, Instructional Preferences, Facilitators and Barriers to Participation

There is very little research that probes into what exactly older people want and need to learn. In Australia, Boulton-Lewis and others (2006) found that older adults believed that their most important learning needs were associated with transportation, health and safety. They were also motivated to learn about leisure activities, and new things such as technology, although with some difficulties due to their lack of background and experience in using technology in their daily lives. 'Young-old' adults were more found to be keener to learn than 'old-old' adults, and their reasons were to keep their minds active and stay mentally stimulated. Villar et al. (2010) found various reasons for older Spanish adults to participate in university programmes. These included remaining active and filling time in a positive way, respite, knowledge motivation and social contact. In Hong Kong, elders were found to be engaged in learning for five main reasons: to meet people, fill up time, learn something new, make life more meaningful and develop personal interests or hobbies (Leung et al. 2005). Others believe that older people need to learn about health management (Kerschner and Pegues 1998; Crane 2001), while some others are concerned about the issue of elders learning about finance (Gregg 1993) and the use of ICT (Stadler and Teaster 2002).

Research also suggests that older people approach learning differently. They may prefer to learn in different ways, at different paces, as well as in different forms. Motivated by different reasons and needs, some elders prefer to enrol in formal and organized courses, while some others prefer to learn by way of informal activities. The Economic and Social Research Council in the UK reported that many older people have in fact engaged in various forms of informal learning through reading, watching educational television and even talking to people (2003). The different needs and motivations for elders to engage in learning suggest that we need to understand the meaning of learning to elders over the course of their lifetimes as it relates to their experiences as learners (Withnall 2000). While there is considerable research on the reasons why elders engage in continued learning, there is no investigation why elders choose not to engage in learning. It is imperative to complete the research literature by understanding why some elders are not participating in continued learning which might be due to a host of barriers that are dispositional, situational and institutional in nature (Cross 1981). Dispositional and situational barriers are related to the individual's personal life and circumstances, while institutional barriers are inhibiting factors presented by policy and support from the government, educational providers and other community agencies.

Manheimer (2009) proposed four new post-career models to highlight the fact that people as they age will want different lifestyles and therefore have differing learning needs and expectations:

1. Neo Golden: pursuing self development and social adaptation associated learning needs: enrichment, socialization and new skills

2. Second career orientation: dream job associated learning needs: learning new skills and new businesses
3. Portfolio life: balance of family, leisure, work and travel associated learning needs: to meet interests, needs and new career skills
4. Continuous employment: extension of midlife career associated learning needs: new skills to keep up for employment purposes

Hence, to plan effectively for elder learning, it is important to understand the learning needs and motivations of the elderly and their reasons for enroling, or more importantly, not enroling, in programmes.

Elder Learning Policy and Provision in Hong Kong

In Hong Kong, the government understands that learning is vital to active ageing and has advocated the benefits of continued learning among the elderly to help improve their health and quality of life as they age. The Hong Kong government endorses the World Health Organization (WHO)'s Active Ageing Policy Framework in which active ageing is defined as 'the process of optimizing opportunities for health, participation and security in order to enhance quality of life as people age' (WHO 2002). The government understands that participation in learning is vital to active ageing and will bring benefits to the elderly to help improve their health and ability to cope with challenges presented by old age. On a variety of occasions, including in policy papers and reports, speeches, and public addresses by senior officials concerned, the government has alluded to the importance of learning for active ageing. For example, in the *Report on Healthy Ageing* (2001) by the Hong Kong Elderly Commission, 'lifelong learning by the elderly' has been identified as one of the four strategic directions for promoting active and healthy ageing among elders in Hong Kong. Also, at the commencement ceremony of the Elder Academy 2008–2009 officiated by the Chief Executive, the Secretary for Labour and Welfare emphasized that pursuing continuous learning enabled elders to keep pace with the times, take part in community service, and continue to contribute to society. More recently, the Financial Secretary announced in his *Budget 2009–2010* the allocation of $10 million to set up the Elder Academy Development Foundation to aim at supporting learning and participation by elders in all sorts of formal and informal educational programmes and activities.

According to the Elderly Commission of Hong Kong, elder learning programmes first emerged in the late 1980s, with most of them organized by non-government organizations (NGOs). This is confirmed by Leung et al. (2005) who noted that learning for older persons in Hong Kong started in 1984. Learning opportunities were mainly provided by elderly care centres and social services organizations, and the courses offered were non-credit bearing and mostly personal development in nature (Zhang and Ha 2001). Examples of these courses include Basic Computer

Usage for the Elderly, Elementary English, Chinese Calligraphy, Water and Ink Painting, Dancing and Tai Chi lessons, etc.

It was also commented by Lee and Chan (2002) that Hong Kong adopted a non-formal approach to elder learning for its elderly citizens in the 1990s. But this changed after the establishment of the Elderly Commission (EC) in 1997. The government since then has taken on a more coordinated approach to elderly policy development with the EC tasked to provide advice on policies and programmes to meet the challenges brought about by an ageing population. As a result, the policy development for elderly education in Hong Kong can be conceptualized as two distinct stages. Stage 1 is pre-1997 and before the establishment of the Elderly Commission, which is characterized by the non-formal approach to elder learning. Stage 2 is post-1997 and after the formation of the EC, where continued learning is conceived as an integral part of healthy ageing and is encouraged by the government in the forms of social campaigns, initiatives and even funding support to providers. Such water-shed development in policies and provisions for elder learning is incidentally marked by the establishment of the Hong Kong Elderly Commission in 1997.

Since its establishment after 1997, the Hong Kong Elderly Commission has been active in initiating many new developments in caring for elders. One most significant development among all is the 'Elder Academy' Scheme launched by the Commission and the Labour and Welfare Bureau in early 2007. With the support of schools and NGOs, 78 elder academies were initially set up in various districts and were well received by the elderly. To date, the network has expanded to include more than 100 EAs in schools and NGOs, plus seven EAs in tertiary institutions. A series of surveys conducted by the School of Professional and Continuing Education of The University of Hong Kong, even before the Elder Academy Scheme was established, shows a rising trend for elders to participate in learning with the percentages of people aged 60–64 participating in continuing education increasing from 3% in 2003 to 12% in 2005 (HKU-SPACE 2006). These figures, however, represent just the tip of the iceberg, and the demand for elder learning should be ever increasing as the ageing population grows. Through the EA Scheme, the government has been proactive in providing funding for education and intergenerational programmes for the elderly. As a result, many initiatives in the form of publicly provided programmes exist, some charging nominal fees, from which elders can choose to learn. The EA Network is expected to grow and expand as continued funding is committed by the government to support provision at various levels.

By way of the Elder Academy Scheme, the government has invited interested education organizations to partner with local volunteer organizations and offer their school campuses for the establishment of elder academies. In the *Application Guidelines of the Elder Academy – Pilot Elder Learning Scheme* issued by the Elderly Commission (2007), elder academies are expected to achieve seven objectives:

1. To promote lifelong learning by encouraging elders to make best use of their time and to keep pace with society through acquiring new knowledge and learning new skills
2. To maintain healthy physical and mental well-being by enhancing their sense of achievement and self-confidence through learning

3. To foster a sense of worthiness in elders by offering a platform for elders to share knowledge, demonstrate creativity, serve the community and continue to make contribution to society
4. To optimize existing resources through partnerships with schools which are equipped with the requisite resources and facilities for learning that can take place after school hours and at weekends
5. To promote integration between the elders and the young by engaging them in learning activities for intergenerational harmony and rapport
6. To strengthen civic education by having uniformed groups such as the Scout Association to offer volunteer services to the elders to promote civic education and to foster community spirit
7. To promote cross-sectoral harmony through collaboration among schools, tertiary institutions and NGOs including District Elderly Community Centres and Neighbourhood Elderly Centres

The approach of operating an elder academy, according to the *Application Guidelines*, is 'a self-help form of learning programme in Hong Kong'. The Elder Academy Scheme is conceived as 'a territory-wide, non-accredited school-based elder learning scheme designed for self-access'. And the plan is to establish one elder academy in each of the 19 districts in Hong Kong. Through joining the scheme, participating schools and organizations will receive a lump sum grant as seed money to establish elder academies, which will operate on a self-financing basis, charging a fee that is affordable for elders who will share part of the cost for financing the scheme. In the scheme, the Elderly Commission and the Labour and Welfare Bureau act as coordinators to encourage cross-sectoral collaboration among schools, non-government organizations (NGOs), tertiary institutions and even a radio broadcaster to work together to promote elder learning. With respect to curricula, the range of offerings can include a variety of both compulsory and elective courses tailored to meet the diverse needs, interests and abilities of elders, with the aim to help raise their standard of living by building up their capability for self-care and adjusting to life in old age. As a result, a wide range of courses are made available, including academic studies and leisure pursuits such as arts, craft and sports. Access to these courses should be barrier-free with no entry requirements and examinations. Upon completion of the study programmes offered by any approved academy, elder learners will be awarded certificates by the Elderly Commission, and a graduation ceremony will be held to congratulate their success.

A Network of 'Elder Academies'

This model of a network of elder academies is claimed to be unique by the Elderly Commission who stated on its official website that it is committed to a 'school-based Elder Academy Scheme with Hong Kong characteristics' (Elderly Commission of Hong Kong 2010). It encourages elders to 'continue learning so as to maintain their physical and mental well-being, foster a sense of worthiness, and promote intergenerational harmony, civic education and cross-sectoral collaboration' through government coordination with schools, tertiary institutions and NGOs by providing some financial support for course offerings. Such cross-sectoral collaborative approach with Hong Kong characteristics sets itself apart from either of the two common approaches of organizing elder learning in many parts of the world. There are generally two major forms of elder learning in Europe with its early development dated back to the 1970s when the University of the Third Age (U3A) was founded in Toulouse, France, with an aim to promote learning in old age. Because of its French origin, this is better known as the French model (Swindell and Thompson 1995), which requires U3As to be associated with traditional university systems. Under the French model, the programmes offered vary widely in content and mode, but usually include lectures and negotiated access to regular university courses, other learning activities and campus facilities. Funding also varies, ranging from university funding, some financial support from the local government, and donations to fees paid by U3A members themselves. The idea of U3A later spread to England in 1981, where it was first established in association with Cambridge University (ibid). However, the concept soon changed with the formation of independent U3As based on local communities where courses were conducted by the members themselves. The self-help approach of the British model is characterized by minimal membership fees; accessible classes in community halls, libraries and private homes; flexible timetables with negotiable curricula and teaching styles; wide course variety and no examinations or entrance requirements. Each U3A is independent and run by its own elected management committee with no government funding (ibid).

The Elder Academy Network in Hong Kong follows neither of these models. The network, claimed to be distinct and unique with Hong Kong characteristics, requires co-investment and joint engagement between the government and various stakeholders, forming a network with a range of schools, institutions, and organizations and developing a multiplicity of offerings, some traditional, some innovatory, some formal, some informal. In order for the network to work effectively, there is a need for clearly defined and effective coordination of interaction, connection and cooperation among and between the wide ranges of providers in such a network of educational provision. There is also a need for support and arrangements for cross sector linkages, easy credit transfer, recognition of prior learning across sectors and boundaries. The idea of networks, as conceived by Chapman (2006), is distinct from traditional forms of grouping of educational organizations and systems, in which hierarchical structures and organizational approaches are most often adopted. The notion of 'network', however, stresses the idea of 'community' as the common element and principle of connection among all relevant stakeholders including the government, schools, institutions, organizations and the participants. Networks, because of cross-sectoral collaboration, have the potential to be more supportive, cooperative, and cost-effective. There is also the opportunity for shared and dispersed leadership and responsibility, drawing on resources and creative efforts in the community beyond those primarily initiated by the government. The relevance of 'networks' as a construct and strategy for the coordination and operationalization of elder learning in Hong Kong is evident in the significant growth and development of a network with over 100 elder academies established within a period as short as 3 years since July 2007.

Future Research and Policy Development

By the work of the Elderly Commission and its sprawling network of elder academies across the territory, the Hong Kong government has, in fact, committed policies and provided financial support and other resources to help providers run courses and programmes for the elders. Through the Elder Academy Network, resources are pooled and expertise and skills put to optimal use to benefit all involved. However, there is limited information as to the effectiveness and impact of such policy and practice on stakeholders. There is a need for research and evaluation to critically review the effectiveness and adequacy of programmes for older adults in the elder academies in schools, NGOs and universities in Hong Kong. Data and views are necessary from the perspectives of policy makers, service providers and elderly learners to evaluate how effective the policies have been in encouraging older adults to engage in continued learning, and to examine why (or why not) elders enrol in the programmes.

A culture of research and evaluation is needed in the interest of developing strong, effective and progressive policy and practice in promoting elder learning in Hong Kong, focusing on the following areas for future conceptual, analytical and empirical enquiry:

- Evaluation of whether current organizational, administrative and financial arrangements through the Elder Academy Scheme are adequate as means of extending and promoting the ideal of education for all
- Stocktaking of existing offerings for elder learning, examining whether they foster or inhibit effective linkages, promote or hinder effectiveness and facilitate participation for and by elders in learning
- Curriculum analysis and evaluation of existing learning provision as a basis for future planning and resource allocation
- Evaluation to improve the network approach to make it more coherent and structured with considerations of quality, standards and expected learning outcomes
- Investigating ways to sustain creative efforts and help mobilize public and private resources to build learning communities for elders by different sectors
- Exploring multi-mode delivery methods of teaching and learning to overcome isolation and difficulties for elders to attend classes
- Addressing barriers to learning by elders and understanding why and why not elders enrol in programmes
- Studying learning practices, processes and provisions, drawing on present good practices for sharing among providers, schools, universities, NGOs and elder learners themselves

Conclusion

This chapter has first described the involvement of older adults in lifelong learning from the East–West cultural perspectives. Second, it has identified and discussed the motivations and factors for elders to engage in learning. Third, it has examined those learning issues considered important for older learners, including their interests, needs, instructional preferences, facilitators and barriers to participation. Fourth, elder learning policy and practice in Hong Kong are outlined to provide the background for the development of a coordinated approach to elder learning by way of a network of 'elder academies' with an aim to pool resources and put expertise and skills to optimal use to benefit all involved. Finally, it suggests that the Elder Academy Scheme be critically reviewed for effectiveness, inter alia, to ensure that it is meeting the needs and expectations of older people and supporting providers in delivering high-quality programmes to elders. To date, no research has investigated the effectiveness of current elder learning policy and provision in Hong Kong or whether the main goal of active ageing through continued learning is being achieved. To determine whether such policy and provision have achieved the desired outcomes, they must be subjected to rigorous evaluation. Only then can these policy and provision claim to have achieved significant and important outcomes for Hong Kong.

References

Ardelt, M. (2000). Intellectual versus wisdom-related knowledge: The case for a different kind of learning in the later years of life. *Educational Gerontology, 26*, 771–789.

Boulton-Lewis, G., Buys, L., & Lovie-Kitchin, J. (2006). Learning and active aging. *Educational Gerontology, 32*(4), 271–282.

Chapman, J. (2006). An analysis of problems, issues and trends in the provision of lifelong learning: lessons learned. In J. Chapman, P. Cartwright, & E. J. McGilp (Eds.), *Lifelong learning, participation and equity* (pp. 317–336). Dordrecht: Springer.

Crane, P. B. (2001). I want to know: Exploring how older women acquire health knowledge after myocardial infarction. *Journal of Women and Aging, 13*(4), 3.

Cross, K. P. (1981). *Adults as learners*. San Francisco: Jossey-Bass.

Dench, S., & Regan, J. (2000). *Learning in later life: Motivation and impact*. Nottingham: DfEE.

Economic and Social Research Council Report. (2003). *United Kingdom*. Retrieved September 11, 2009, from http://www.esrc.ac.uk

Glendenning, F. (2001). Education for older adults. *International Journal of Lifelong Education, 20*(1/2), 63–70.

Gregg, D. W. (1993). Financial gerontology. *Journal of the American Society, 47*(2), 32. Retrieved from the ABI = INFORM Global Database (Document ID:284197).

Hammond, C. (2002). What is it about education that makes us healthy? Exploring the education-health connection. *International Journal of Lifelong Education, 2*(6), 551–571.

Hammond, C. (2004). Impacts of lifelong learning upon emotional resilience, psychological and mental health: Fieldwork evidence. *Oxford Review of Education, 30*(4), 551–568.

Jarvis, P. (2001). *Learning in later life: An introduction for educators and carers*. London: Kogan Page.

Kerschner, H., & Pegues, J. M. (1998). Productive aging: A quality of life agenda. *Journal of the American Dietetic Association, 98*(12), 1445–1448.

Kim, K. H. (2004). An attempt to elucidate notions of lifelong learning: Analects-based analysis of Confucius' ideas about learning. *Asia Pacific Education Review, 5*(2), 117–126.

Lee, W. O. (1996). The cultural context for Chinese learners: Conceptions of learning in the Confucian tradition. In D. Watkins & J. Biggs (Eds.), *The Chinese learner: Cultural, psychological and contextual influences*. Hong Kong, Japan/Melbourne, Australia: Cooperative Education Research Centre and Melbourne/The Australian Council for Educational Research.

Lee, P. W., & Chan, K. M. (2002). *Development of lifelong learning among Hong Kong new generative elderly: Abstract of final research report* [In Chinese]. Paper presented at the Hong Kong Young Women Christian Association on 16 March 2002.

Leung, A., Lui, Y. H., & Chi, I. (2005). Later life learning experience among Chinese elderly in Hong Kong. *Gerontology and Geriatrics Education, 26*(2), 1–15.

Lu, L., Cooper, C. L., Kao, S. F., & Zhou, Y. (2003). Work stress, control beliefs and well-being in Greater China: An exploration of sub-cultural differences between the PRC and Taiwan. *Journal of Managerial Psychology, 18*(6), 479–510.

Lussier, R. N. (2005). *Human relations in organizations* (6th ed.). New York: The McGraw-Hill Companies.

Manheimer, R. J. (2009). *New paradigms for old: Trends and developments in later life learning in North America*. Retrieved 7/24/09 from: http://www.lancaster.ac.uk/depts/conted/AEAconference.htm

McClusky, H. Y. (1971). *Education: Report for the 1971 White House Conference on Aging*. Washington, DC: U.S. Government Printing Office.

Merriam, S. B., & Mohamad, M. (2000). How cultural values shape learning in older adulthood: The case of Malaysia. *Adult Education Quarterly, 51*(1), 45–63.

Narushima, M. (2008). More than nickels and dimes: The health benefits of a community-based lifelong learning programme for older adults. *International Journal of Lifelong Education, 27*(6), 673–692.

O'Connor, C. M. (1987). Elders and higher education: Instrumental or expressive goals? *Educational Gerontology, 12*, 511–519.

Ross, C. E., & Mirowsky, J. (1999). Parental divorce, life-course disruption, and adult depression. *Journal of Marriage and the Family, 61*(4), 1034–45.

Rowe, J., & Kahn, R. (1999). *Successful aging*. New York: Random House.

Ryan, J., & Louie, K. (2007). False dichotomy? 'Western' and 'Confucius' concepts of scholarship and learning. *Educational Philosophy and Theory, 10*(11), 405–417.

Schuller, T., Preston, J., Hammond, C., Brassett-Grundy, A., & Bynner, J. (2004). *The benefits of learning: The impact of education on health, family life, and social capital*. London/New York: Routledge Falmer.

Silverstein, N. M., Choi, L. H., & Bulot, J. J. (2001). Older persons on campus. *Gerontology & Geriatrics Education, 22*(1), 13–30.

Stadler, K. M., & Teaster, P. B. (2002). Aging, nutrition, technology, web sites, older people. *Journal of Nutrition Education and Behavior: Nutrition Education and Older Adults, 34*, S67–S68.

Stine-Morrow, E. A. L., Parisi, J. M., Morrow, D. G., Greene, J., & Park, D.C. (2007). An engagement model of cognitive optimization through adulthood. *The Journals of Gerontology: Series B Psychological sciences and social sciences Special Issue 1: Cognitive Interventions and Aging, 62B*, 62–69.

Swindell, R., & Thompson, J. (1995). An international perspective on the University of the Third Age. *Education Gerontology, 21*, 429–447.

The Elderly Commission of Hong Kong. (2001). *Report on healthy ageing*. Hong Kong: Hong Kong Government.

The Elderly Commission of Hong Kong. (2007). *Elder academy pilot learning scheme application guidelines*. Hong Kong: Hong Kong Government.

The Elderly Commission of Hong Kong. (2010). http://www.elderlycommission.gov.hk. Accessed July 31, 2011.

The School of Professional and Continuing Education of The University of Hong Kong (HKU-SPACE). (2006). *Survey on the demand of continuing education in Hong Kong 2005/2006*. Hong Kong: HKU-SPACE.

Valenzuela, M. J. (2009). *It's never too late to change your mind*. Sydney: ABC Books.

Villar, F., Triado, C., Pinazo, S., Celdran, M., & Sole, C. (2010). Reasons for adult participation in university programs in Spain. *Educational Gerontology, 36*(3), 244–259.

Withnall, A. (2000). *Older learners – issues and perspectives* (Working Papers of the Global colloquium on supporting lifelong learning). Milton Keynes: Open University. Retrieved March 14th, 2009, from http//www.open.ac.uk/lifelong-learning

Withnall, A. (2006). Exploring influences on later life learning. *International Journal of Lifelong Education, 25*(1), 29–49.

World Health Organization. (2002). *Active ageing: A policy framework*. Geneva: World Health Organization.

Zhang, W. Y., & Ha, S. (2001). *An investigation into the learning attitude, motivation and preferences of the older adults in Hong Kong*. A paper presented for the 15th Annual Conference of the Asian Association of Open Universities hosted by India Gandhi National Open University, New Delhi, India.

List of Authors: Biographical Details

Short Biographical Notes

Biographical Details of Contributors to this Volume

Richard G. Bagnall is Dean (Research) for the large and diverse Arts, Education and Law Academic Group at the Nathan Campus of Griffith University, Australia.

Simon Biggs is currently the Brotherhood of St Laurence, Professorial Fellow and Professor of Gerontology and Social Policy at the School of Social and Political Sciences, University of Melbourne. He was formerly Professor at the Institute of Gerontology, King's College, London, UK. He has researched and written extensively about social theory, social policy and ageing.

Roger Boshier is Professor of Adult Education at the University of British Columbia in Vancouver. From 1984 onwards he has been studying adult education in China and, more recently, the national learning initiative. He has published articles about K'angta, the Yan'an War College built after the Long March, Lushan, the "Learning mountain" in Jiangxi, innovative educational projects in Zhabei, Hangzhou and elsewhere. He is interested in "foreign devil" adult educators active in China from the 1920s onwards. His most recent article is entitled "Hey There Edgar Snow, What Happened to the Red Star over Yan'an?" From the 1980s onwards he directed the UBC Adult Education Diploma programme in Hong Kong.

Gillian M. Boulton-Lewis is an Emeritus and Adjunct Professor, in the School of Design at Queensland University of Technology in Brisbane. She has made a significant contribution to research in learning and education across the lifespan and in a range of areas. She is currently involved with research programmes in early childhood and ageing. Her work demonstrates a deep interest in how people learn.

G.M. Boulton-Lewis and M. Tam (eds.), *Active Ageing, Active Learning: Issues and Challenges*, Education in the Asia-Pacific Region: Issues, Concerns and Prospects 15,
DOI 10.1007/978-94-007-2111-1, © Springer Science+Business Media B.V. 2012

Laurie Buys holds a Ph.D. in Human Rehabilitation and a Graduate Diploma in Gerontology from the University of Northern Colorado. She is a Professor in the School of Design, Faculty of Built Environment and Engineering at Queensland University of Technology. She is National Immediate-Past President of the peak professional body, the Australian Association of Gerontology. She is Board Member of the Centre for Subtropical Design and a member of the Brisbane City Council's Inclusive Brisbane Board. She has over 60 refereed publications covering her research interests which include active ageing, ageing and intellectual disability, social sustainability, green buildings, high density living and community engagement.

Ernest Chui is Associate Professor in Social Work and Social Administration at the Hong Kong University. He is also currently the Director, Sau Po Centre on Ageing at the same university. He has undertaken research on residential care, housing needs, long term care, poverty, financial needs, health and other issues affecting the elderly in Hong Kong.

John Field is a Professor in the Institute of Education, University of Stirling, Scotland, where he directs the Centre for Research in Lifelong Learning. He has written widely on lifelong learning; his book on Lifelong Learning and the New Educational Order (Trentham 2006) is a standard point of reference in the field. He has also written on social capital, active citizenship and voluntary activity, as well as on the social history of adult education and training, and he recently completed a secondment to the UK's Government Office for Science, where he helped to co-ordinate an international study of mental capital and well-being. He is currently directing a major research project, funded by the Economic and Social Research Council, on learning, identity and agency across the life course.

Evonne Miller is a social psychologist and Senior Lecturer in the School of Design at Queensland University of Technology. Evonne has over 30 refereed publications, covering her diverse research interests in social gerontology (active ageing, quality of life, physical activity), social sustainability (sustainable buildings and communities) and behaviour change (sustainable lifestyles, public acceptability of controversial technologies). She is also the Queensland President of the Australian Association of Gerontology, Australia's largest multidisciplinary professional association of people working in the diverse fields of ageing.

Nancy Lloyd Pfahl is an adult educator and lifelong learner whose primary research interest is narrative learning. Since 2004 she has worked independently in Washington, DC as a consultant and researcher. In 2003 she served as US Community College Consultant to Indonesia, working with local officials to adapt the education model to four locations. Previously in Illinois she served as Chief Development Officer at College of DuPage, one of the largest community colleges in the USA. During her 15-year tenure she collaborated with faculty, staff, and community members to initiate and develop more than 600 learning initiatives funded for more than $85M US dollars.

Rick Swindell is a teacher, researcher and practitioner in the field of lifelong learning and successful ageing. He has played a leading role in the development of the self-help model of the University of the Third Age (U3A) within Australia and internationally. He is cofounder of U3A Online, the world's first virtual U3A, which harnesses the talents of retired experts to write and teach online courses for older learners from many countries. In 2004 he was admitted as a Member of the Order of Australia for services to later life education.

Maureen Tam is Associate Professor in Elderly Education in the Department of International Education and Lifelong Learning at the Hong Kong Institute of Education (HKIEd). She is also Deputy Director of the Centre for Lifelong Learning Research and Development in the Institute and concurrently Academic Coordinator of the HKIEd Elder Academy. Her recent research interests are elder learning and active ageing and she holds a HKIEd Internal Research Grant to conduct a critical international review of the state of theorization, policy and research in elderly learning and education.

Index

G.M. Boulton-Lewis and M. Tam (eds.), *Active Ageing, Active Learning: Issues and Challenges*, Education in the Asia-Pacific Region: Issues, Concerns and Prospects 15, DOI 10.1007/978-94-007-2111-1,

MIX
Papier aus verantwortungsvollen Quellen
Paper from responsible sources
FSC® C105338

If you have any concerns about our products,
you can contact us on
ProductSafety@springernature.com

In case Publisher is established outside the EU,
the EU authorized representative is:
Springer Nature Customer Service Center GmbH
Europaplatz 3, 69115 Heidelberg, Germany

Printed by Libri Plureos GmbH
in Hamburg, Germany